LOVING, SUPPORTING, AND CARING FOR THE CANCER PATIENT

LOVING, SUPPORTING, AND CARING FOR THE CANCER PATIENT

A Guide to Communication, Compassion, and Courage

STAN GOLDBERG

ROWMAN & LITTLEFIELD
Lanham • Boulder • New York • London

Published by Rowman & Littlefield
A wholly owned subsidiary of The Rowman & Littlefield Publishing Group, Inc.
4501 Forbes Boulevard, Suite 200, Lanham, Maryland 20706
www.rowman.com

Unit A, Whitacre Mews, 26-34 Stannary Street, London SE11 4AB

British Library Cataloguing in Publication Information Available

Library of Congress Cataloging-in-Publication Data

Names: Goldberg, Stan, 1945- author.
Title: Loving, supporting, and caring for the cancer patient : a guide to communication, compassion, and courage / Stan Goldberg.
Description: Lanham : Rowman & Littlefield, 2016. | Includes bibliographical references and index.
Identifiers: LCCN 2016012440 (print) | LCCN 2016023989 (ebook) | ISBN 9781442266155 (cloth : alk. paper) | ISBN 9781442266162 (Electronic)
Subjects: LCSH: Cancer—Patients—Care—Popular works. | Caregivers—Popular works.
Classification: LCC RC263 .G62 2016 (print) | LCC RC263 (ebook) | DDC 362.19699/4—dc23
LC record available at https://lccn.loc.gov/2016012440

♾️™ The paper used in this publication meets the minimum requirements of American National Standard for Information Sciences—Permanence of Paper for Printed Library Materials, ANSI/NISO Z39.48-1992.

Printed in the United States of America

This book is dedicated to my beautiful granddaughter Mattea, who I hope with other people of her generation will find this book irrelevant and ask "What was cancer, Grandpa?"

CONTENTS

ACKNOWLEDGMENTS

I use "loved one" as an umbrella term for family and friends and "he" and "she" interchangeably to help the writing flow. While all stories are true, names, gender, age, and locations were changed to protect privacy. Quotes are based on my recollections or notes made shortly after an interaction. Thanks to my many clients and patients who invited me into their lives for thirty years and shared their fears and joys. Without your courage this book would not have been possible.

Thanks to Kimberly Cameron, whose commitment and faith in the purpose of this book got it into the hands of Suzanne Staszak-Silva and the Rowman & Littlefield Publishing Group.

1

THE BASICS

At least once in your life, a loved one or friend will say to you, "I have cancer," and when you hear these three words, you may struggle with a response. If loved ones or friends haven't informed you of a cancer diagnosis, they will. Every year fourteen million people worldwide learn they are living with or may die from this disease, and the number of people living with cancer trends upward as new medical breakthroughs extend life.[1] Almost twenty years ago a good friend informed me of her breast cancer. I wasn't sure what to say, so I uttered the most commonly used phrase whenever someone shares terrible news: "I'm so sorry." I always wished my response had been more useful. It took years of my serving people with cancer and being the recipient of "I'm so sorry" responses to my cancer before I could become more helpful.

Cancer can attack any organ in the body, pop up at unexpected times and places, steal nutrition from healthy cells, destroy lifelong plans, and create general havoc for those living with the disease and their community. Scientists have accumulated vast amounts of information on the diagnosis and treatment of cancer, but the literature lacks specific suggestions for what to do or say when people reveal their diagnoses. The purpose of this book is to share the knowledge provided to me over the past thirty years by loved ones, friends, clients, and patients. Think of the eighty-three section headings (e.g., Reduce the Chaos of Cancer) as *what* you should know about cancer or your loved one. But knowing what to do is not the same as knowing *how* to do it. At the end of each section are suggestions for how to implement the information you just learned. There are 266 suggestions for taking you from compassionate intent to helpful behaviors. In the Appendix all of the "whats" and "hows" are listed. Every suggestion comes from research, my experience with cancer, and what my clients and patients have

1

told me helped them. Think of the suggestions as the cumulative knowledge of what cancer patients would like to happen. Not everything in this book applies to everyone. Think of them as cafeteria offerings where you get to choose. Take what you find useful and disregard what doesn't apply. The material contained in this book is not a theory of how people should treat those of us living with cancer. Rather, these are observations of what people living with cancer found to be helpful.

REDUCE THE CHAOS OF CANCER

A cancer diagnosis makes life chaotic. The disease acts as if it is an improvisational musician capable of changing direction without notice. Our body, with the help of radiation, surgery, or drugs, defends against the disease as it mutates and grows. Just like the uncertainty a jazz tune's direction will take, cancer's development winds through our life in expected and unforeseen ways. There are some things we do know: when the cancer first started showing diagnostic indications, the dates treatment will begin and end, how soon after chemotherapy hair falls out, and the survival statistics for our type of cancer. While the "known" facts of a cancer journey create anxiety, the intensity of this feeling pales when placed against what we don't know such as, will there be pain? Will drugs be sufficient to stop the pain? Will I live beyond the number of expected years (i.e., five-year survival data)? How will my family and friends react to my disease? Will I lose significant parts of my life even if I survive? Will I be able to cope with or adjust to the changes I'm about to experience? These questions and a host of others keep us awake at night.

It would be nice if our path would be similar to a well-laid-out city grid pattern, where the street numbers are sequential or run alphabetically from "A" to "Z." You always know where you are by reading the street signs. If I'm crossing Sixth Street, the next street will be Seventh. Unfortunately, our travels are more like a country-road adventure where directions from a local are fuzzy: "Go down a ways until you come to the big rock on the left, then the road you're looking for is a piece down the road. Look yonder for the biggest sycamore tree, and take a soft left." Directions such as these lack the comfort of hearing "Go down to Forty-Third Street, turn left, and go for two blocks until you come to Madison. Turn right and 785 Madison is on your left." Disappointments, ecstasy, and revelations will fill the country-road journey you are about to take with your loved one. It promises everything found in a spellbinding novel but unlike a book, you can't close it when you've had enough. Expect more chaos than stability on the journey.

Suggestions

1. Expect a cancer journey to take an uncertain path.
2. Don't underestimate the psychological effects of uncertainty.

ASSUME THE WORLD OF YOUR LOVED ONE DIFFERS FROM YOURS

In a small restaurant north of San Francisco, I overheard a woman complaining to a friend about the ingratitude of a relative diagnosed with breast cancer. "I don't understand it," the woman said. "I tried to be helpful. Isn't that what you do for family? I told her of the wonderful new supplements I read about on the Internet; things to control her cancer. She almost bit my head off when I offered suggestions. I mean, these weren't off-the-cuff recommendations. Some came from Dr. Oz. They might save her life. You'd think she'd be more appreciative." The woman tried to be helpful and probably was compassionate, but she didn't understand her relative entered a different world after receiving a cancer diagnosis. Her agenda of "health through better nutrition" was something her relative who faced an uncertain prognosis didn't want to hear. Cancer, either stable or progressive, shapes almost all experiences. The presence of a life-altering disease affects people in more ways than cancer-free people may understand. It often becomes evident when a cancer-free person argues with a friend or loved one his interpretation of what they both experienced was not accurate or an overreaction. It's a problem of different perceptions, not honesty.

The changes in perceptions caused by illness or disease were evident when I was at San Francisco State University and treated a young woman who had a stroke. Difficulties in processing information remained after she recovered her speech and language. What had been fulfilling interactions, such as having an intimate conversation with someone in a crowded room, became confusing. The types of words were no different than those spoken at social events she attended before the stroke, but her ability to understand them in the presence of noise was impaired. To someone who didn't know she had had a stroke, this was the same person they had always known and loved. "Maybe I should wear a sign," she said, "something like 'my brain is fried.'" She told me her friends didn't understand the cognitive changes the stroke caused. She walked without any paralysis, seemed to under-stand everything, and spoke with the same eloquence she had before the stroke. They couldn't see the stroke's effects, so they didn't modify their expectations of what their friend was capable of doing. They would choose favorite restaurants, and because they were considered "happening places" they were noisy. Noise for my client meant it would be an evening of confusion, frustration, and humiliation. She would look at someone who was speaking, smile, nod her head, and have no idea what the person was saying. The experience was devastating. Her stroke, just as cancer does, changed her world.

Even knowing someone has cancer doesn't sensitize people to the changes the disease causes. A patient struggled to hold on to short-term memory as his brain tumor grew. He could keep a multitude of dates in his mind before cancer. With the cancer's progression, even writing down the dates didn't help since he forgot to look at his calendar. When a relative who knew of the diagnosis chastised him for forgetting a birthday party, he realized how few people could understand his new world. The philosopher, Merleau-Ponty, wrote about the futility of believing reality is objective. We see the world, according to phenomenologists, through a complex array of filters that distort emotions, feelings, and events in ways consistent with each person's values and needs.[2] The distorting effects of these filters become evident when we crunch information into something going beyond observations.

Imagine two people asked to listen and evaluate Thelonious Monk's *Bright Mississippi*,[3] which is described by one reviewer as "an idiosyncratic, complex, unpredictable, occasionally noisy, always compelling foray into improvisation."[4] The first listener is in his seventies and grew up in a small midwestern town. He believes the traditional values guiding his life are under attack. *Bright Mississippi* for him is a series of random, discordant notes representing everything wrong with current society. The second person is a professional jazz musician in her thirties who lives in New York City and relishes progressive values and change. She listens to the same cut and hears an incredible tune embellished by dynamic chords. The music is emblematic to her of an exciting new world of progressive values in which she believes. *Bright Mississippi* for her represents the future. The same mu-sic, but different perceptions. Think about disparate interpretations of the Thelonious Monk cut as you try to understand your loved one. It doesn't make sense to talk about an independent reality that's the same for both of you. A unique perspective on life comes from living with a potentially terminal disease. Within those of us living with cancer is a cluster of angry cells whose only purpose is to kill us. People can read about death, and even care for someone with a terminal prognosis, but unless they experience the possibility of dying, everything is a theory.

Suggestions

3. Don't allow your agenda to prevent the use of compassionate behaviors.
4. Take the perspective of your loved one who is living with cancer rather than your own.
5. Don't evaluate a loved one using your perspective.

HONESTLY EXPRESS YOUR FEELINGS

A cancer journey involves both the mind and the heart. If you find it difficult to express emotions think back to the time when you were a child. You approached the world without being defensive. You hadn't learned yet to protect yourself, but as you grew, you believed in the importance of developing defensives, resulting in the creation of a personal armor. These defenses often stay with us long after their utility ends. For example, a teenager rejected by a love interest experienced such intense pain that he remained guarded for years. When he needed new defenses, they joined existing ones. Layer upon layer formed as he aged. He believed that with enough defensives he could be protected from most hurtful situations. But as medieval warriors paid a price for the protection of chain mail and overlapping metal plates (limited movement), not letting go of useless defensive mechanisms is also costly (not able to be emotionally honest). You expressed feelings as a child, without caring whether someone perceived you to be vulnerable. If you loved someone, you stated it (e.g., I love you Daddy). Something didn't look right, you weren't afraid to call attention to it (e.g., What's that thing on your face, Grandma?). Someone's comments or unskillful behaviors hurt and you expressed your pain (e.g., I don't like it when you tease me).

Throughout the cancer journey, your willingness to be open and honest will be important to your loved one, but it will require shedding your defenses as I did clothes as a child in Eastern Pennsylvania. My mother would prepare me for the frigid winter temperatures by bundling me in layers. First was the flannel pajamas, followed by corduroy pants and a wool shirt. Then came the sweater, jacket, and "un-losable" mittens with a string extending from one sleeve to the other. The layers were important for surviving the bitter cold but unnecessary in a warm house where my mother peeled off each layer. The same applies to expressing emotions. Strip away the defensive layers and you'll not only experience something important but will better serve your loved one's needs.

Suggestions

6. Express your feelings about your loved one's cancer.
7. Don't expect your loved one to share her feelings if you can't share yours.
8. If you have difficulty expressing feelings, start with how children experience the world.
9. The past is the source of most defensive mechanisms—you don't need them in the present.

CHANGE COMPASSIONATE THOUGHTS INTO HELPFUL BEHAVIORS

How do you define compassion? Defining it involves the same problem cited in a 1964 Supreme Court ruling on obscenity. For the majority opinion, Judge Potter Stewart wrote:

> I shall not today attempt further to define the kinds of material I understand to be embraced within that shorthand description ["hard-core pornography"], and perhaps I could never succeed in intelligibly doing so. But I know it when I see it.[5]

As with pornography, we know compassion when we see it. One popular definition of compassion comes from the Vietnamese Buddhist priest, Thich Nhat Hanh.[6] He said envision the person in need as if she is your mother—the person who nursed and protected you when you were helpless. "Compassion" for Thich Nhat Hanh is what you would do for your mother. Others define compassion as what we do to fill our hearts with love.[7]

We hope the ability to be honest about one's emotions and willingness to express them is enough to transform compassion into helpful behaviors, but it's not. A step between compassionate thought and helpful behaviors is necessary.[8] The missing step involves knowledge of *how* to be compassionate. Imagine planning a trip from New York City to San Francisco. You're unfamiliar with the routes, so you go to the local travel office and say to the clerk, "How do I get to San Francisco from here?" She points west and says, "That way." The direction is correct, just as an open heart is necessary for compassion to develop. Pointing west may not be enough for the traveler to arrive in San Francisco in a reasonable amount of time. Compassion may not be enough to help a friend or loved one living with cancer.

The missing step involves not only the *how* of transitioning from intent to useful behaviors but also how the cancer is changing your loved one's life. Think of the relationship between the two as similar to what a person must do to jump over a ten-foot span, one hundred feet off the ground. He might run fast, jump high, and hope he lands on the other side. Best case scenario is he lives. Worst case, well, we know what can happen. Those of us old enough to witness the motorcycle jumping of Evel Knievel in the 1960s and 1970s were amazed by his feats.[9] We were transfixed by the dramatic buildup and waited to see whether he would survive. Unknown to us was that his jumps over cars, buses, and canyons were based more on the physics of movement than being daredevil tactics.[10] His knowledge enabled him to live. He moved from intent to a behavior through understanding physics. Throughout Knievel's life, there was a focus on action. It's interesting that this high school dropout's philosophy of life paralleled that of the brilliant mathematician and humanist Jacob Bronowski. Bronowski believed the world could be grasped only by action, not by contemplation.[11] I think the same is true for compassion: If you want to convey compassion to your loved one or friend don't express it only through words; use concrete actions. You need to *do* something, not just *think* about it. There's a story of a young man who came to a monastery hoping to learn the secrets of life from an enlightened old monk. After being there one year, he was allowed to ask the master one question.

"Master, what is the secret of life?"

"Have you eaten your rice gruel?" the old man said.

"Yes," the confused student responded.

"Then wash your bowl."

The monk left and never spoke again to the student. In the monk's mind, after revealing the secret of life was in "doing," not "thinking," he didn't need to say anything else. We should do the same to express our compassion. Don't worry about selecting the most appropriate words or responses.

Sometimes words are sufficient but can be subject to misinterpretation. After hearing "I'm so sorry for what you're going through," a client said, "If I hear that phrase one more time, I'll scream." She didn't question anyone's sincerity, but rather the condolences became a string of words losing strength since no actions followed. Yes, continue to say compassionate words, but accompany them with actions. We think of compassion as something that can produce wonderful results for people on the receiving end. Compassion not only benefits the person receiving it but also the person giving it. It's analogous to Shakespeare's line in *The Merchant of Venice*.

> The quality of mercy is not strain'd,
> It droppeth as the gentle rain from heaven
> Upon the place beneath: it is twice blest;
> It blesseth him that gives and him that takes.[12]

Suggestions

10. Compassionate thoughts are not sufficient to be helpful. You need to transform them into behaviors.
11. You will need to understand your loved one's world before you can change compassionate thoughts into helpful behaviors.
12. Be prepared to do acts displaying compassion.
13. Your compassion will be a gift to both you and your loved one.

RECOGNIZE REACTIONS TO CANCER DIFFER

Everyone comes to cancer with a personal history of experiences, values, fears, and preferences. A personal history shapes how we deal with cancer. Someone who is accepting may view his cancer as another facet of living. A religious person might believe her cancer is a test from God. A problem solver might delve into every aspect of cancer's treatment as if it were a complex puzzle. The personal contexts of people with cancer are as varied as personalities. The context of my cancer made it difficult to be honest about my feelings. Cancer wasn't an illness found in my family's genes, and I knew few people who were living with it or had died from it. I was a university professor in the area of speech-language pathology for almost thirty years. My training and profession emphasized observation, understanding, and constructing strategies for solving problems.[13] And emotions? They were interfering factors I kept in check as a professional. That was my context. Cancer would be another interesting clinical problem to solve: no more challenging than determining why a five-year-old didn't develop language or identifying appropriate language strategies for someone who had a stroke or creating a set of activities enabling a stutterer to speak fluently. The approach I used to deal with my cancer came from how I acted professionally and personally. The first of many mistakes I made was using an email to inform family and friends—other than my wife and adult children—about the diagnosis.

Hi, Folks,

First the good news. My latest poem, "Tidal Movements," received 2nd place in a national poetry/photography contest sponsored by the American Society on Aging and the National Council on Aging. I attached it here. The poem was generated by a canoe trip Rich and I took in the Everglades. It's about accepting aging and not dwelling on it. I'm convinced first place went to a picture of a prune. All this stuff is a setup for the _____ in the subject line of this email.

I have prostate cancer. I thought it would be easier just telling everyone at the same time. It looks like the cancer is confined within the prostate gland. Therefore, the probability of it having metastasized is very low. If I have surgery, it probably will be no earlier than the second week in June after Wendy begins recovering from her hysterectomy (I believe that's called a gotcha! line). We'll be cranky with each other, confined to bed, and Justin, who will be home for the summer, will play nurse. If I opt for radiation, the procedure will begin shortly. I still have two more expert opinions to get.

So how are the poem and cancer connected?—attitude. I'm convinced the body/mind relationship can play a big part in preparation for and recovery from things like cancer. I feel very good about what I can do for myself and the positive effects it will have. If nothing else, what a great topic for a new poem or magazine article! For a title "Me and My Prostate" and a picture of me holding the gland in my hand, smiling at it.

Get the picture? No gloom, no doom. While I have been regularly meditating, I plan to become consistent and increase my practice. Goodbye fat, fried foods, red meat and other things associated with cancer. Time to lose weight and exercise regularly. So if you see me thinner and buffed out, its not the result of cancer. I'm finally doing something about my health. Funny isn't it, how the thought of death makes you take your health more seriously?

Love you all and take care,
Stan

I reread this email thirteen years after I wrote it, and memories of desperation and fear returned. I faced an uncertain prognosis and struggled with deciding how and to whom I should reveal the diagnosis. My words were upbeat, sometimes comical, and I viewed a life-threatening disease as a puzzle in need of a solution. A few people complimented me on keeping a "stiff upper lip" and creating a positive email. What they didn't understand was the joviality of the email was an attempt to hide the terror I experienced. My analytical approach created a barrier between my emotions and what I would be facing. Years later, a few friends confided in me that they heard the fear in my words and were distressed that they didn't know how to help.

Everybody reacts to a cancer diagnosis differently. We hear the word "cancer" and a multitude of visions surface. When I heard the word, I associated the diagnosis with loss, diapers, and a premature death. The oncologist told me I had an "80 percent probability of living at least five years," but I focused on the 20 percent probability of dying. Some people I counseled reacted as I did to hearing they had cancer. Others were as honest about their fears as I wish I had been thirteen years ago. A woman whose friends said "she wore her heart on her sleeve" was forthcoming in sharing the diagnosis with family, friends, and even casual acquaintances. She didn't fall apart as her friends predicted but rather developed coping strategies. The more in touch a person is with her emotions, the more likely she will share the diagnosis. Wearing "my heart on my sleeve" would have been a better approach than the "problem-solving" one my life history dictated.

You don't need to know your friend's past to understand her context. Think about how she reacts to events having a strong emotional component. Does she shy away from talking about anything difficult, or does she face it? Does she express concern when someone is in need or does she pretend it doesn't exist? How amenable is she during arguments to seeing other people's viewpoints? By analyzing her reactions to difficulties, you can construct a useful picture of her context. Context becomes a means for predicting attitudes and behaviors and the basis for understanding differences in how you and your loved one perceive the world.

We would like to believe a joint experience is consistent—what you and your husband see is the same. How we view an event often has more to do with our needs and history than our notions of objective reality. One powerful example of the distinction between perception and objectivity is *Rashomon*, the 1950s movie Akira Kurosawa wrote and directed.[14] It is the story of a samurai's gruesome death. The audience members, as the "objective" viewers, watch the drama unfold, believing they know what happened. In court, the event is described by four people who witnessed it: a woodcutter, a priest, the deceased samurai's wife, and the bandit who killed the samurai. The four saw the same event; yet each gives a different description of what happened, and each believes his or hers is the honest rendition. None of their accounts are close to what the audience members saw in the film. The scenes created by Kurosawa from their testimonies could have come from four different events. Discrepancies such as these often occur when two people are involved in the same event but whose history and needs are different. It's similar to how you and your husband may view the effects of his disease.

The discrepancy between what happened and what we think happened becomes distorted at least twice. The first when it occurs and the second is when we remember it. We don't store events in our memory as an objective occurrence. Just as Kurosawa's characters did, we store it through perceptual filters. When we retrieve them, we don't even bring forth the original distortion. According to current research on memory, whatever is stored is again changed; parts drop out, and new distortions are added.[15] We think of our mind as if it is a computer, but the brain doesn't fact-check the way a computer does. You write an email to a specific address, and your Internet server "decides" whether to accept or reject it. You receive one of two messages: "email sent" or "no such address." The feedback is simple—you typed the address correctly, you typed it incorrectly, or the address no longer exists. Nothing is quite as straightforward when the brain processes information. For example, your wife says, "You aren't sensitive to my needs. You never listen." Your brain compares the incoming information to its stored memory. "Aha!" the brain says. "She's being manipulative again." Your past interactions and memories can distort a straightforward expression of an emotion. When you attempt to retrieve the interaction, it will again be distorted: information will be dropped out, and other information changed to be in line with what you thought happened. Consistency between your needs and what you thought happened trumps truth.

In the eighteenth century, philosophers spent countless words arguing about "truth" and "reality."[16] Some believed there was only one reality. Others maintained truth was relative since everybody sees the world differently. While that discussion was academic, the importance of understanding why people may see things differently has real-world consequences. The next time you are in an argument with your loved one and you begin to evaluate her words and behaviors in absolute terms, remember, you're looking at it through a set of distortions. To some extent, we all are actors in *Rashomon*.

Suggestions

14. How your loved one reacts to emotional events is a blueprint for how she will respond to a diagnosis of cancer.
15. An emotional reaction to a cancer diagnosis by your loved one is better in the long run than a "stiff-upper-lip" attitude.
16. Accept your loved one's version of the facts instead of arguing about them.

WHY IT'S NOT A BATTLE

Those of us living with cancer often are the recipients of accolades such as "You're so brave in your battle with cancer" or "You should be proud you are a survivor." These compliments and many similar ones come from the heart and are meant to make those of us living with cancer feel special. They are positive statements applauding the efforts we make living with a killer disease. I always feel uncomfortable when I'm the recipient of the compliment, yet I smile and say, "Thank you." Your friend may be placed in an untenable position if cancer is treated as a battle. If she "beats" cancer, she's a heroine, someone who won against stacked odds. But what if she can't control the cancer? Some people who are fighting against the disease and losing question whether they are trying hard enough. I served people whose "fight" was lost from the moment of the diagnosis.[17] Survival statistics for some types of cancer are encouraging if the cancer is found in the early stages. Identification during the later stages shows decreased survivorship.[18] And then there's the timeline. The majority of survival statistics are limited to five years. That doesn't mean people don't survive for more than five years; rather the studies lasted for only five years.

Despite a patient's positive attitude, ingestion of multiple supplements, and adhering to her physician's suggestions, her Stage IV breast cancer couldn't be controlled. For the first few months following the diagnosis, her symptoms were minor. She and her friends were buoyant. They were going to "beat" it, and high fives were abundant. Six months after the diagnosis, it was apparent her cancer was spreading despite chemotherapy and radiation. By structuring her relationship with cancer as a battle, she began thinking she was at fault for losing the fight. I met her in hospice when I was a bedside volunteer. She was overwhelmed with guilt, believing the cancer had come back because she hadn't tried hard enough, even though she had followed all medical and spiritual recommendations. Worse than self-doubt was her fear that her friends were disappointed with her effort, although they had never said anything disparaging about her relapse. They were supportive, but she still wondered if they blamed her for the cancer's reoccurrence. She was despondent during the last few weeks of her life, not because she was dying, but rather because of the guilt she carried for not having fought hard enough.

We're not heroes. We live our lives as you do. Living with cancer involves a mix of denial, acceptance, and adaptation. There are days when I want to give up and others when I pretend my precancer energy is still there. And on my most realistic and best days, I adapt my behaviors and expectations to my reality. I never just survive—I adapt. Adapting is different from surviving or giving up. It is an active process where I look at what I'm facing and determine whether I'm capable of still doing it. If I am, I proceed. If I'm not, I make adjustments. I was touched when a friend who knew I could no longer fly-fish alone in the wilderness offered to take me to a "fish and pay" park, where stocked fish almost hooked themselves on your line. He knew it would not replace the fishing experiences I no longer have because of the cancer but rather that it was an attempt to help me adapt to the loss.[19]

Living with cancer in many ways is like swimming in a riptide. Try to move back to shore against the tide and you won't progress. Most likely, the tide will continue pulling you out to sea. Swim across the current, and you'll be released. That's what people do who live with cancer. We meet the illness every day, confronting problems and often allowing the experience to teach us what's important in life. We don't survive; we adapt. "Surviving" is a rigid concept. One either survives or dies. There isn't much room for equivocation. Adaptation involves a constant adjustment to circumstances. It requires an active engagement between the person, her disease, and the positive things that can be done to enjoy life. Focus on how your loved one is adapting instead of placing him on a pedestal. Compliment him on how he adjusts, modifying activities as needed and accepting limitations.

All people with cancer must decide how they will confront the disease. Some people become passive, giving up on any active involvement in treatment. They allow medical personnel, friends, and family to decide everything about intervention. Their passivity may be the result of believing they don't have enough information, having given up, or placing all power in the hands of a superior being. Others may view their journey as if they are ranchers, bringing the herd together and moving the cattle down the road. Some see the battle in a religious context, with the forces of good fighting against the forces of evil. Others conceive of the fight against cancer as a mind-body conflict. Regardless of how we view cancer, we meet it every day as if it were an annoying relative who at times makes our life difficult while at other times wants to take us out for a beer and teach us something about life.

What happens when you and your husband view the journey differently? You see it as a battle while he relies on a mind-body relationship. In John Lennon's 1970s hit song, *Whatever Gets You Through the Night*, he sings about the importance of using whatever works in dealing with life.[20] The message of the song is many paths can lead to the same destination. Accept the approach your loved one chooses even if it's one you don't like. Painful decisions may be necessary if you want to be supportive. Even if you think the battle will be lost and your husband views himself in a life and death struggle, support his beliefs. Few certainties exist with cancer. A reversal or even a new drug on the horizon could improve his condition. But if neither happens, help him focus on aspects of his disease where success is possible, as was the case with a woman with lung cancer. Her life revolved around social justice causes, from civil rights to combating sexism. She was joyful knowing through her efforts inequities might change, and she applied the same values to dealing with her cancer. From the time she woke in the morning and put on her "battle clothes" (knit cap and bib overalls), her fight began. She ingested medications, took supplements, and prepared cancer-fighting foods, envisioning her body's healthy cells attacking the cancer. Despite her best efforts, her cancer progressed. Her adult daughter, who idealized her mother, was distraught seeing her losing to the cancer. She could accept her mother's eventual death, but witnessing daily failures was painful. She introduced positivism into her mother's life by encouraging her to become involved in activities with a high probability of being successful, such as attending a party in the evening or spending time walking in the neighborhood. These "minigoals" replaced the less achievable goal of defeating the cancer. The daughter couldn't prevent her mother's death, but she was able to provide her with successful experiences. She never stopped battling, right up until she died.

Living with cancer can involve a series of defeats and negative experiences. Regardless of the severity of the disease, you can structure win-lose activities to increase the chances of success. One of the easiest ways is what the daughter in the previous example did: She chose a simple, small activity (e.g., attending a party for a short time) rather than one so big that the likelihood of success was minimal (e.g., defeating the cancer).

Suggestions

17. Don't compliment us on being survivors.
18. Compliment us on learning how to live with cancer.
19. Accept how your loved one views her confrontation with cancer, regardless of what you believe.
20. Focus on small, winnable conflicts with cancer rather than ones involving survival.

WHAT YOU WILL EXPERIENCE

We've all had the painful experience of wanting to help friends and family and not knowing how to do it. Sometimes it involves minor issues, but often they are gut-wrenching ones, as was the case of a man whose contact with his sister was sporadic. They talked once or twice a month on the phone and visited each other two or three times a year, despite living less than ninety miles from each other. He was a legislative analyst residing in Sacramento; she was a software designer for a startup in San Francisco. Most of the time, the sister initiated contact, so when she called, her brother assumed it was the monthly phone call where both would catch up on each other's lives and utter pleasantries.

"Hi," she said, and then continued with, "I have cervical cancer." He thought it was the worst news anyone could have delivered, until she said, "and it's untreatable." She lived alone having recently split with her partner. The brother remembered their mother's cervical cancer and knew his sister would need 24/7 care within a month. He took a leave of absence and moved into her small apartment. They were close throughout their lives, yet he stumbled when faced with transforming compassion into helpful behaviors. He knew as her condition deteriorated she would need help in everyday activities, such as food preparation and personal hygiene, but he didn't know how to approach these issues with her. *Should I assume she needs help, or should I wait until asked? When is the time right to discuss how I feel about her? What can I say to ease her journey? Is she afraid of dying?* He assumed his compassion would be easy to actualize, but it wasn't. Compassion for him required more than "being present" and using kind words. He needed to convert compassion into useful behaviors. He tried doing it by placing himself in her shoes. He asked himself, "If I were in her position, what would I want?" He answered the question based on *his* experiences and values, not his sister's needs.

We may attempt to "simulate" a loved one's condition, but everything is conjecture until you experience a life-threatening diagnosis. Alfred Korzybski, the linguist, wrote, "The map is not the territory."[21] While his field was general semantics, his wise thought applies to understanding the world of someone living with cancer. We can never know what it's like for a loved one to live with a potentially lethal disease. We can speculate, and if you experienced a serious illness, you might come close. But with everything that goes into an emotion, you'll still miss it. At a workshop the Buddhist priest Sogyal Rinpoche related a story told to him.[22] A social worker was counseling a man who was dying. She asked him if it was important that people he interacted with understood what he was going through. The man responded, "No, that's not possible. But I want them to act as if they do."

In everyday interactions you will find examples of the difficulty in transitioning from thought to action. I saw a visually impaired man in New York City waiting for a traffic light to change before crossing the street. The corner had a ramp, but the man positioned himself over a portion of the curb undergoing repair. He would stumble when the light changed. I saw two people looking at him who appeared to be contemplating whether to say or do anything. I came to his side when neither moved to help and explained he would fall if he continued. I asked him if he would like me to guide him to the ramp and offered my elbow as we crossed the street. He was grateful for the information and the offer. After we crossed the street, he again thanked me and said, "You know, I often bump into things knowing people are around me and don't say or do anything." I asked why he thought they were reluctant to offer help. "I think many don't know how to react to someone who is blind. I know most are compassionate, but they don't know how to express it or are afraid I'll take offense." Six months later in downtown San Francisco, I saw an example of someone who knew how to move from compassionate intent to a helpful behavior. He leaped out of his sidewalk restaurant chair when a person in a wheelchair wasn't able to continue on the sidewalk because of an obstruction. In listening to their conversation, I heard him say his cousin was disabled and he knew how difficult it was for someone in a wheelchair to maneuver through obstacles. The New York City example involved not knowing how to respond to a disability. The San Francisco one emphasized how knowledge can shape responses.

Not everyone possesses the knowledge of the San Francisco man when he encounters a situation requiring transitioning from intent to action. Often, lessons on how to be helpful come from new situations, as it was for me when my wife had a stroke caused by a heart arrhythmia. Overnight, my daughter and I became 24/7 caregivers. My wife recovered with no lasting disabilities, but the three-month experience left me with a new and deeper understanding of long-term caregiving. Addressing the physical needs of a loved one with a chronic or terminal illness is difficult enough. Factoring in your emotional needs and those of your loved one can be mind boggling. There will be times when you will struggle between satisfying your loved one's needs and your own, as I had to do with my wife for three months. I realized it was necessary to subvert my needs to hers, but I couldn't help experiencing some resentment. It was an irrational emotion I was ashamed of having, since I did (and still do) love my wife and knew my needs were trivial compared with hers. You may develop similar guilty feelings—the same ones experienced at one time or another by most caregivers.

Suggestions

21. You will experience feelings of helplessness.
22. You can place yourself in your loved one's shoes, but don't expect to get it completely right.
23. You are not God. You will make mistakes.
24. Don't feel guilty about satisfying your needs.

THINKING ABOUT CANCER IS NOT THE SAME AS EXPERIENCING IT

Everything you imagine about a potentially lethal disease is a theory until experienced. Sometimes your thoughts are right on, but often, such as with me thirteen years ago, my idea of what it would be like to have cancer wasn't close. "You have prostate cancer," the urologist said. He continued speaking while I tried getting past the shock of his words. "And it's aggressive." I don't remember what I said to him, but I still become nauseated thinking of the four words. I was fifty-seven, and death was theoretical—something that happened to people of my parent's generation. I was a full professor at San Francisco State University and involved in research and publications. Life was good. And death? Well, it was something beyond my horizon, something I saw in movies and read in novels. Something I would "eventually" experience. With the four words, "You have prostate cancer," *eventually*, turned into *now*.

I searched the Internet and found one in seven men develop prostate cancer.[23] The exclusivity of the group made me think of Groucho Marx's reaction when he received a telegram from an exclusive Hollywood club offering him membership. He wrote back, "I don't want to belong to any club that will accept me as a member."[24] Just as Groucho reacted to his invitation, I wasn't thrilled to become a member of the "Men with Prostate Cancer Club." Groucho had the option of declining; I didn't. My discomfort continued when I read the five-year survival rates. Most men around seventy diagnosed with prostate cancer survive at least five years and usually die from other causes.[25] I was fifty-seven and intended to live more than five years. I also read men with prostate cancer that was confined to the gland had a 100 percent survival rate. I didn't know whether my cancer was in the gland or had proliferated. If I chose surgery, the surgeon couldn't determine whether it had spread until he removed the gland. If I chose radiation, the metastasis would be undetectable until tumors grew in other parts of my body. The bad news continued with my Gleason score.[26] The Gleason score is a combination of PSA (protein specific antigens) and the aggressiveness of the cancer cells. My PSA was 16 (normal is less than 1.3),[27] and the urologist described the cancer cells as "aggressive." My Gleason score was an ominous 7. I had read that Frank Zappa, the noted rock musician who died from prostate cancer, had a Gleason score of 9, one less than the maximum. My score was closer to his than a "5 or lower" Gleason score, with encouraging survival statistics.[28]

I wrestled with how to tell to my wife and two adult children. What words would I use? Should I use humor to soften the blow, or should I pretend the diagnosis had the significance of a cold? *Hi, Dear. I'm grilling steak for dinner. Sorry, it's not done yet. I was delayed starting the grill because the urologist called and told me I have prostate cancer. What would you like for dessert?* No, my nonchalant approach wouldn't work, nor would my usual way of dealing with emotional issues, which was to become "professorial." I approached life as a complex clinical problem needing objective solutions. *Here is problem A. Try using B, C, and D. If none of them work, try E, F, and G.* A ridiculous approach to something terrifying. I thought about the unskillful things I did throughout my life and wondered whether I had time to apologize. Would I have the courage to admit my mistakes, no less ask for forgiveness? What about my long list of goals? Could I complete them, or should I begin arranging them in order of importance? If prioritized what criteria should I use—importance to me, importance to my family, importance to my profession? Would my life change in unacceptable ways if I survived?

Throughout my life, I was an avid outdoors person. I still viewed myself as "young," despite the many infirmities of middle age. *After all, cancer doesn't happen to young people. Well, maybe not many. I'm fifty-seven, for God's sake! That's not old enough to get cancer, right?* Images of being debilitated by the disease went through my mind as if it were a preview for a horror movie. I had been self-reliant my entire life and rarely asked my family or friends for help in doing anything physical. I thought back to the time when my friend told me she had cancer. Now, I would be saying the three words to my family. I wondered what went through her mind when she informed me of her diagnosis. Did revealing the diagnosis shatter her world as much as I anticipated the words would affect mine? My world changed with four words, and I didn't know how to deal with the diagnosis. I couldn't predict the changes but knew the greatest would involve my identity: the old Stan, who existed before the diagnosis, would be replaced by someone I didn't know.

Suggestion

25. Thinking about cancer will not give you the type of understanding derived from experiencing it.

REDUCE STRESS AND TAKE CARE OF YOUR NEEDS

We often impose a "Mother Teresa" mantle on ourselves and experience guilt for taking care of our needs. You might develop resentment as I did if your needs are continually subverted to those of your loved one. Your life is changing. You may have sacrificed a career, ended social relationships, and become consumed with the care of your loved one. You never cease observing, worrying, and waiting for something to happen as a primary caregiver. The stress is overwhelming and tests your capacity to provide compassionate care. What you will experience is analogous to a bucket with a hole. As long as incoming water doesn't exceed the amount going out, the bucket will never overflow. Increase the flow of incoming water or narrow the opening of the hole, and water spills everywhere. Spilled water is like stress. Assume that as the length of time involved in caregiving increases or a loved one's needs increase, the flow of emotions and physical demands will also increase. However, the hole—your threshold of effective caring—can be widened by taking regular breaks, walking, sleeping in an adjoining room, or anything producing emotional or physical rest. Don't feel guilty about going for a walk, attending a theater production, laughing at a movie, or reading a novel in the next room while someone is caring for your loved one. I often hear the lament, "I don't have the time to reduce my stress." While there are many proven methods to reduce stress, one of the easiest is meditation.

Meditation is an effective form of stress reduction not requiring much effort or time.[29] There's nothing magical or religious about it. Rather, it's a psychological exercise allowing the mind to declutter itself, to get rid of negative lingering thoughts and stop anticipating future events. Almost before one thought leaves, six more arrive: what you did yesterday, what you will do tomorrow, how you could have done something better the day before. These thoughts and hundreds of others take up your concentrative ability, making it harder to stay in the present—the time frame necessary for providing the best care for your loved one. Recent neuropsychological studies have shown that meditation can change physiological responses and reduce anxiety.[30] In other words, meditation can strengthen your ability to deal with what you face as a caregiver. Think of meditation as a giant broom sweeping away useless thoughts interfering with your ability to provide compassionate care.

The more you declutter your mind, the easier it becomes to focus on the specific activities you are doing. Nothing complicated about that. Children not yet concerned with the past or future are proficient at staying in the moment. How often have you focused on something in the present to the exclusion of the past or future? You may be listening to your husband describe something related to his cancer while wondering whether the groceries you purchased yesterday (past) will be sufficient to create an acceptable dinner tonight (future). How would your reactions change if you were able to listen to his concerns without thinking about the past or future? Some years ago, I conducted an informal study trying to identify whether there were traits outstanding clinicians had in common.[31] One characteristic feature I found was the ability to listen and respond to clients as if only they existed. The clinicians ignored their problems before going into the therapy room and until the session ended, put aside nontherapy concerns. For these great clinicians, only the client existed for the next sixty minutes. It's a model you may wish to emulate with your loved one.

Some people who try meditation complain it didn't make any difference after their first, second, or third session. With no miraculous results, they abandoned it and went back to accepting stress as a part of life. What they didn't realize is that the effects of meditation and most forms of stress reduction are cumulative. Think of a garden ignored for months whose plants are overgrown with weeds. The nutrients necessary for keeping your lettuce and strawberries were gobbled up by the unwanted plants. Every day you pull out some weeds and wait for the vegetables and fruits to recover. Meditation works in a similar manner. After a few weeks of consistent practice (e.g., fifteen minutes twice a day) your ability to focus on caregiving activities will increase.

Some caregivers view taking time to reduce stress as selfish. That was my opinion when I canceled my attendance at an all-day flute session after my wife had her stroke. What I failed to realize is the reduction of my stress would benefit not only me but also her. Many of the caregivers I counseled also felt guilty when they thought about taking time for themselves. After all, it is their loved one who needs care, not them. There is no need to feel you're selfish since stress reduction not only calms your mind but will help you be more alert and efficient. Your stress reduction is a gift for your loved one.

Suggestions

26. If you don't reduce stress, your ability to be compassionate and helpful will be reduced.
27. Although there are many ways of reducing stress, meditation can be used when the time is short and caregiving help is minimal or nonexistent.
28. Do a stress-reduction activity twice a day, for fifteen minutes if possible.

2

REVEALING A
CANCER DIAGNOSIS

Your friend's needs and expectations of how you will react will deter-mine whether she shares the diagnosis or keeps it a secret. The person with cancer sees who she is and compares it with who she may become. The changes can look frightening. Those of us living with cancer believe our body betrayed us, and we may be grappling with our place in a new and frightening world. When someone says, "I have cancer," she is not only revealing a medical condition but also inviting you on a journey that hopefully will end with a remission or cure.

Compassionately listening to the dreadful news is only one of many things you'll find necessary to be helpful. It will also be important for you to be supportive by offering specific help rather than being general. You may be forced to balance hope with the reality of a terrible prognosis. Your loved one's trust in you will be tested on small and significant issues, rang-ing from being on time to the difficulty of keeping the diagnosis a secret. After your loved one learns of his diagnosis, he may experience emotional shock so debilitating you may need to help with decisions. People living with cancer have different personalities and backgrounds and are at vari-ous points of acceptance. The uniqueness of our situation warrants unique responses.

THE DECISION TO REVEAL A CANCER DIAGNOSIS

I no longer thought about death in theoretical terms when I received an uncertain cancer prognosis. Death became something real and frightening. What I thought a distant event—my death—might be lurking around the corner. Instead of years to address my regrets and complete my goals, time may be limited. The decision to share my diagnosis was momentous because it was a statement of vulnerability. It's not only the thought of death from cancer weighing on us but also the journey we are about to take. For some, it involves only minor annoyances, but for others, there's painful chemotherapy, radiation, or surgery. Treatment can irrevocably change some lives. Others will wrestle with interventions only prolonging the inevitable. It is from within this world that we struggle with the decision whether to reveal the diagnosis. Saying "I have cancer" is a statement of what we may be facing and a test of our trust in you.

The decision to share the diagnosis isn't a big deal when the cancer involves only minor lifestyle changes. Your loved one's physician may have informed him the cancer is treatable and shouldn't disrupt his life. A friend with a reoccurring skin cancer was told to stay out of the sun, apply a special cream, and visit the dermatologist for a chemical facial burn once every six months. The doctor made his recommendation fifteen years ago. Little changed in my friend's life, and since his cancer is less interfering than a seasonal cold, few of the suggestions in this book are appropriate for him. Changes in the lives of others are more dramatic. We struggle whether to reveal our condition or bear our new status alone.[1] We may crave support, but our needs are tempered by concerns such as *What will he think of me? Will she still love me? Will they pity me? Will I be treated as if I'm the disease?*

Every person living with cancer is an amalgam of values, beliefs, experiences, needs, and desires. Even if our physician minimizes what we might face as he treats the cancer, we're probably familiar with adverse reactions to the intervention. If ignorant of them, an Internet search will supply horrible stories based on some facts, much hearsay, and hand-me-down "wisdom" bearing little resemblance to the truth.

Suggestions

1. Saying "I have cancer" is an invitation to participate in what may be a long journey.
2. View the sharing of a cancer diagnosis as an honor.

BE CAREFUL ABOUT USING LABELS

A diagnosis of cancer has the potential for stigmatizing, and nobody wants his disease to define him. The use of a label ("cancer survivor," "cancer victim," etc.) to describe a person is onerous, but the use of labels is an established shortcut way of identifying a particular problem. For example, "aphasic," "Alzheimer's patient," "cognitively impaired," "developmentally delayed," and "language disordered" are terms people commonly use withoug even thinking about the implications for the person living with the problem. A friend or loved one living with cancer hears "cancer victim" or "cancer survivor" and may believe the person using the term views her as the disease.[2]

Most people—including me—take the shortcut approach and use a label rather than a more precise description such as "a person who suffered a stroke," "a patient with Alzheimer's," "a person dealing with a cognitive impairment," "a child with language delays," or "a loved one coping with cancer." Some people say even though they know the disease doesn't define the person, it's easier using an abbreviated term rather than a more accurate, but longer, one. There are two negative consequences of using labels that outweigh the time saved by not using a more accurate description. The first is the person who is labeled may wonder whether the speaker can see past his cancer. A client whose prognosis was good became annoyed when his relatives referred to him as a "cancer victim." His oversensitivity led him to believe they were ignoring other aspects of his life, such as "runner," "CEO," "father," and "husband." Whether the relatives thought of him as a label is questionable. Of importance was his perception. The second reason to avoid labels is that studies of language usage found the repeated usage of certain words or descriptions can solidify how a person is viewed.[3] Whenever possible, try not to use labels even if you see your loved one or friend as a complete person.

Suggestion

3. Don't treat the person living with cancer as if he is the disease.

BE SUPPORTIVE AND SPECIFIC

There is an awkward moment when people hear someone is living with cancer or, worse, expects to die from it. Listeners hear "cancer," and they become silent as if struggling to find the right words to say. I came to realize listeners' responses to illness and death often come from their level of comfort with end-of-life issues. Despite the desire to say or do the right thing, listeners often feel paralyzed. I know I did when my friend told me she had cancer. After telling her how sorry I was, I reacted as most people do, by offering help through the use of generalities such as "If there's anything I can do, please call" or "When you need something done, please let me know." The rationale for being general is to allow your friend to contact you for a variety of needs. By keeping offers general, we assume our friend will add the specifics when needed. This belief leads to misinterpretations of compassionate intentions. A patient said to me that he questioned family members' sincerity when they offered to help since they never went beyond generalities. The offers were always "If you need anything, please call." He interpreted the relatives' offers as disingenuous. "If they wanted to help," he said, "why didn't they offer to do things they knew I couldn't do anymore—like cooking meals and cleaning?" His energy level dropped with the radiation treatments, making it difficult to do even the easiest tasks. Despite needing help, he didn't contact his relatives. Some relatives attributed the lack of contact to his not needing help. Others were confused.

An example of how to be specific is, because you know chemotherapy causes exhaustion, you could say, "I know shopping for food may be difficult for you. I'll pick you up tomorrow morning at 10:00 and we'll do it together." A friend who was having chemotherapy for a controllable form of cancer told me that walking after the treatments was better than sitting. I said, "What time would you like me to come over after your treatment next week?" She said with little hesitation, "11:00 a.m." She understood my desire to help was genuine rather than something "socially appropriate." I wanted to help, and my specificity made my intent clear. Specificity also increases the likelihood that your friend will accept help since you may not know what she needs or the type of help she will accept. A "no, thank you, but I'm grateful you asked," is better than your friend believing you are inconsiderate. Don't be afraid to be too helpful.

Your loved one's decision to ask for and accept help may be the acknowledgment that he is beginning on an unpleasant path. I wasn't able to do many physical things when I was recovering from prostate surgery. I rarely called my adult son for help, even knowing moving a lightweight box or picking up a few pieces of lumber would cause pain. Was I acting rationally? Of course not, since I was aware everyone's offer to help was genuine and heartfelt. But asking for help meant I was accepting how the cancer was changing my body. I wasn't ready for the changes and persisted in doing everything myself for three months until I realized the changes were permanent at best, progressive at worst. Make a list of your loved one's daily activities if you're not sure what to offer. Nothing complicated, but be specific. For example, you know he wants to pay bills every Friday but often feels too tired by midday. Offer to take on the responsibility. The effects of cancer or its treatment can result in a loss of energy, pain, physical discomfort, or "fuzzy thinking," among other things. Your list of activities should begin with waking in the morning and end with going to bed. Circle those you believe may require your assistance and ask your loved one for confirmation. You'll be amazed how easy it will be to list activities for which you can offer help.

Acceptance of a dependent relationship can be difficult for many people if independence is an important part of their identity, as it was for a client.[4] Before her divorce, she had relied on her husband for most things during their twenty-five years of marriage. After their divorce, she was forced to live independently. It was difficult at first, especially taking care of financial matters. Gradually, what was frightening became the best part of her life: independence. But independence was the first thing she lost following chemotherapy for breast cancer. Among other problems, she couldn't lift grocery items from her shopping basket into her car. She didn't call her best friend to take her shopping. She was willing to struggle rather than admit she needed help. You can do two things if you believe your friend needs help but is reluctant to ask. The first is be supportive. Often the reluctance is an attempt to preserve a precancer image. The second is to help her accept a changing life. Asking for help may be dependent on accepting what goes with a cancer diagnosis. I engaged in inappropriate activities until reality (strained muscles) told me I was becoming a different person. Once I accepted my new identity, I had no problem asking my son or anyone else for help.

Your loved one's cancer is not static.[5] The disease may progress, stall due to the treatment, maybe even lie dormant for months or years. But changes are likely, and with each change, his needs will adjust, as will activities you'll need to do. He will be joyful when he can say, "I'm okay. I can do that by myself now," but be prepared if the cancer moves in a less positive direction. He can't ignore the cancer's progression when he loses abilities he once thought unassailable. Don't be afraid to ask for guidance since you may not be able to keep up with the changes. While some changes may be so gradual, they are difficult to notice, others can be dramatic. A simple statement such as "Do you need help with answering your emails today?" is better than assuming either he does or prefers to do it by himself. In *The Teachings of Don Juan,* Carlos Castaneda asks, "Does this path have a heart? If it does, the path is good; if it doesn't, it is of no use."[6] The journey you are on with your loved one is 80 percent heart and 20 percent head.

Suggestions

4. Be specific regarding what you're offering to do.
5. Your loved one may be rejecting your help not because she doesn't need it but rather because accepting help acknowledges the effects of cancer.
6. Make a list of your loved one's daily activities. Then ask her for input on how you can help.
7. The repeated rejection of help may require a discussion of how the cancer is changing your loved one.
8. Cancer is dynamic, and what you got right today may be wrong tomorrow.
9. It's preferable to be overhelpful than to underestimate your loved one's needs.

BALANCE HOPE WITH REALITY

Those of us living with cancer often hear phrases such as "Let's hope for the best" or "Don't worry, everything will be fine." We know you say the words with the best of intentions and a compassionate heart. We want to believe your rosy prognosis, even when logic and facts say our cancer is formidable. Your expressed hope can be the only thing positive in a miserable day, week, or month, but your support doesn't require hoping for a cure. Often, the most supportive action can be the quiet acceptance of what we are experiencing. A client who had been optimistic about her multiple melanomas became depressed as various treatment options were exhausted. Near the end of her journey, she told me the most positive event since developing cancer was her husband holding her hand during a debilitating chemotherapy treatment. Living with cancer doesn't require a sugar coating, and often the delusion can make adapting more difficult. A client who knew her husband's lung cancer was terminal kept saying to him, "There's hope." Her reasoning was her husband would be devastated if he knew he would dead within months. She believed not telling him was her final gift. He understood the severity of his disease and concluded that his wife was not sensitive to what was happening to his body.

Inappropriate expressions of hope not only come from friends and family but also professionals who treat cancer. Medical personnel assured me new eradication treatments would be available before my prostate cancer became uncontrollable. I kept waiting for the magic bullet during the first few years following the diagnosis, hoping a cure was on the horizon. Thirteen years after the diagnosis, I still receive emails from friends about new "miracle" cures, ranging from natural supplements to abandoning all meat products. I know they believe the news will be uplifting, but it rarely is. Warmed-over, untested beliefs are touted as miracle cures, and others, amenable to scientific research, won't be available until years of clinical trials are completed. People coping with other cancers tell me about receiving similar emails from well-meaning friends and family. One patient with terminal bowel cancer said he was encouraged by his Internet chat room friends to try a controversial surgical and radiation procedure almost guaranteeing miraculous results. Website testimonies by people "cured" of similar cancers touted the surgeon's approach. He was jubilant, believing his death sentence was lifted. Up until the time of the surgery, attempts by his partner to help him prepare for dying were rebuffed. One week after surgery and radiation, the "miracle" cure proved to be a scam for duping desperate people.

There are various reasons people with cancer believe the implausible claims of both well-meaning individuals and disreputable scammers. Many of them think they didn't accomplish enough in life. Others need time to "correct" unskillful behaviors, and a small number fear what will happen after they die. These reasons can make a person gullible, as it did a research scientist in the 1970s who was diagnosed with an inoperable brain tumor. Mainstream physicians told him they could do nothing to stop the tumor's growth. However, alternative medicine practitioners and opportunistic marketers pushed laetrile injections.[7] Laetrile clinics proliferated in Mexico to administer a modified form of amygdalin, a naturally occurring substance found in the kernels of apricots, peaches, and almonds. The research scientist understood the importance of data but ignored their absence in assessing the wild claims made by the drug's manufacturer and the Mexican dispensing clinic. His justification for choosing an unproven treatment was the same many people receiving a terminal diagnosis say, "What do I have to lose?"

Most medical and research personnel studying cancer are skeptical about treatment approaches lacking data. People who believe in alternative approaches without data cite the famous line by the astrophysicist Carl Sagen, "The absence of evidence is not the evidence of absence."[8] They are implying alternative intervention protocols may be effective even without testing. It's an argument holding little value for scientists, but one giving hope to people living with cancer. It also becomes a marketing tool for unscrupulous entrepreneurs.

Don't assume your friend fell for a scam if he chose an unproven alternative therapy. I have followed what I call a "shotgun approach" for the past thirteen years, ingesting supplements, following dietary guidelines, exercising, and having intermittent ADT (androgen deprivation therapy). Substantial evidence for the effectiveness of my treatment choices exists for only the slower growth of tumors following hormone injections.[9] Data regarding supplements, diet, and exercise are less clear.[10] Despite thinking of myself as a clinician who always seeks objective data, I embrace supplements, diet, and exercise, whose acclaimed positive effects are yet to be proven. I tell friends who question my use of unproven treatments that the use of alternative approaches is acceptable if they do not produce adverse consequences and are not a substitution for an established protocol. When I discuss my treatment choices lacking efficacy, I think about the 1930s comedian, W. C. Fields. He was a lifelong atheist, and according to a popular story, when he was close to death a friend found him reading a Bible. "Bill," his friend said, "you're an atheist. Why are you reading the Bible?" Fields looked up from the book and said, "Looking for loopholes."[11]

I believe most people living with cancer search for loopholes—including me. The desire to continue living makes your loved one vulnerable to well-meaning but unscientific advocates of treatment protocols as well as unscrupulous peddlers of hope. Be supportive when you can—not because you believe in a miracle—but rather because that's what your friend needs. Don't stop with support; become a detective. Start with the US Food and Drug Administration (FDA.com), the most informative source on drugs and treatment protocols.[12] On its website, you will find four categories of information:

- Information on FDA-approved brand name and generic drugs
- Index to drug-specific information
- MedlinePlus: Consumer drug information from the National Institutes of Health
- Medication guides information

If you can't find what you need on the FDA website go to the websites for the American Cancer Society, M. D. Anderson Cancer Center, National Cancer Institute, National Breast Cancer Foundation, or any other legitimate organization. Find the source of the unapproved treatment protocol. It will most likely be the Internet. Scour the site for research citations and read them. Become suspicious if there is no research but an abundance of personal testimonies. Often typing in "Scam" followed by the treatment protocol will reveal complaints about the product or program. Despite everything you did to change your loved one's mind, he may still choose an unproven treatment. Instead of trying to convince him it's worthless, offer a compromise: criteria both of you can agree on to determine whether the approach is working. For example, if there is an improvement, you will support his choice of protocols; if not he will resume using an established treatment.

You may find yourself in the uncomfortable position of supporting his tragic mistake as many critics thought happened with Steve Jobs's choice of treatment for his cancer. His biographer, Walter Isaacson, wrote that Jobs declined surgery for a form of pancreatic cancer whose survival statistics were high with early treatment.[13] Instead, he chose unproven alternative methods. Whether his choice shortened his life is uncertain, but many in the scientific community viewed it as a poor choice.[14] Given the intellect of Steve Jobs, it appears something other than logic was important in his decision to decline a proven intervention protocol. Don't be too hard on your loved one, if he is choosing hope over logic.

Suggestions

10. Don't be a cheerleader.
11. Limit hope to achievable goals.
12. Don't inundate your loved one with news of miracle cures.
13. Withhold your unqualified support for treatment protocols lacking data.
14. Support alternative approaches if the protocol isn't a substitution for one with data.
15. Visit FDA.com or other reputable websites if you think a treatment protocol is a scam or worthless.
16. Negotiate objective criteria for ending a treatment's use.

THE PROFESSIONAL MANAGEMENT OF CANCER

Before the 1960s, it was routine for physicians to withhold terminal diagnoses.[15] Today, their willingness to discuss unfavorable prognoses has improved. Medical ethicists speculate that the reluctance to discuss end-of-life issues is generated from doctors' discomfort. They are trained to prolong life, relying on heroic efforts and expensive interventions if necessary to accomplish one goal—the extension of life. Some critics even maintain that the decision not to tell a patient of a terminal diagnosis has more to do with ego than with ethical practice. Physicians counter that not telling patients of a terminal diagnosis extends life. The belief, however, is not supported by data, leaving the practice questionable at best.[16] Physicians' reluctance to be straightforward about the prognosis can stem from other issues including whether the patient or family wants to know. The neurosurgeon who operated on my brother-in-law held the longevity and emotional stability position. He ignored the need my brother-in-law had for getting his life in order. Withholding the prognosis did not increase my brother-in-law's life span (he died within the limited survivability range for glioblastomas), and it limited the time he had to prepare for death.

The ethical concerns about withholding a terminal prognosis have received increased attention in the medical community.[17] Most people agree that withholding a terminal prognosis is unethical. The debate now centers on how to provide the information. Should physicians withhold a terminal diagnosis from an aging parent if family members request it? Is it ethical for a doctor to shade the information so it's less traumatic to the patient? When should the physician tell a patient the prognosis is terminal? The debate raises more questions than it provides answers. Ask your loved one's physician for straightforward answers regarding her approach to conveying information to terminally ill patients. A client maintained that his wife had only a mild form of cancer since her doctor never said it was terminal. His and his wife's belief in the authority and wisdom of the medical community was absolute. If the physician didn't use the term "terminal," they chose to believe the wife's cancer was curable and assumed they had years to discuss end-of-life issues. Both refused to acknowledge her condition until just before she slipped into a coma.

A preference for the unvarnished version of my cancer is why I prefer realistic supporters rather than cheerleaders. The playwright Jean Anouilh said, "I like reality. It tastes like bread."[18] It's the view of cancer I've held since being diagnosed with the disease. Confrontations between delusion and reality rarely lead to anything positive. A woman confided in me as her husband's cancer progressed that he become more adamant the condition was temporary. He insisted his "feeling poorly" would turn around in a few weeks. She tried explaining to him that he wasn't getting better and discussions should focus on end-of-life issues. For three months they argued. She kept presenting him with undeniable facts that his cancer was progressing. He found an explanation for each to mitigate the prognosis. Worse, he believed his wife was looking forward to not having him around, even accusing her of planning an affair with one of their friends. Eventually, he accepted his mortality, not because his wife's insistence wore him down, but rather because he was ready.

I told my current oncologist I don't want him to be a cheerleader. He said in response, "My goal is to keep you alive as long as I can while preserving the quality of your life." His heartfelt words were a mix of compassion, understanding, and reality. I know if my cancer becomes un-controlled, he won't be afraid to begin the conversation many physicians try to avoid about whether to continue life-extending treatment. We have an inherent need to be hopeful in the management of cancer. The blissful fantasy that a cure is around the corner, at least for me, does not last for more than a few hours. The reality of living with cancer returns with each new hot flash, unexplained emotional lability, transient bone pain, and speculation whether I'll be around to teach my granddaughter to fly-fish.

I'm not alone in experiencing the reoccurring fear that cancer will outwit modern science. In conversations with people whose cancer is ac-tive, in remission, or "cured," they often say, "What if they didn't get all the cancer?" or "What if the dormant cancer cells become active?" The concerns come from people who have completed their treatment protocol and those who have lived cancer free for twenty years.[19] We hope terrible things will go away or end. We hope we won't lose a loved one. We hope for so many good things that we try to transform beliefs into facts, think-ing optimism is compassionate. Your loved one's smile is so intoxicating when she believes her condition will improve; you may ignore reality, not wanting to think about the devastation that will occur when declines in her health crush hope. You may wonder what the harm is in telling her she will survive. Shouldn't you want this for her? Shouldn't you want your positive thoughts to take away the dread of what this disease can do? Yes, but your assessment of the cancer's strength shouldn't be based on optimism, nor should optimism be tied only to survivability.

You can attach optimism to day-in, day-out activities rather than sur-vival as a caregiver did whose wife had Stage IV uterine cancer. Through-out their five-year journey, both believed she could control the cancer. They both became realistic when her cancer became virulent. Her physi-cian was clear—at best, she had months to live. For the husband and wife, optimism changed from believing in a cure to day-to-day functioning. Both were optimistic she would be over her nausea by 1:00 p.m. when they were to visit friends. It was a simple goal and one worth rejoicing about when nausea ended. Both were optimistic they could walk in the evening before dinner, a triumph worth celebrating by uncorking a vintage bottle of Chardonnay. They scaled back time references to minutes as the cancer progressed. Close to her death, he focused on small goals such as finishing a spoonful of soup. Their days were filled with optimism until she died.

Suggestions

17. Honor your loved one's views regarding the reality of her prognosis.
18. Confine your optimism to the successful completion of small events, not the defeat of cancer.

BALANCING HONESTY WITH COMPASSION

Our minds often do a balancing act with the truth on one side and necessity on the other. An example is the "butcher's thumb," a common practice before prepacked meats became available in the 1960s. The butcher would place his thumb on the edge of the scale while weighing a piece of meat, adding a few ounces to the total. He knew what he did was wrong but justified the dishonesty with an economic pressure argument: "A few pennies won't make a difference to my customers. At the end of the month, it can mean the difference between keeping my shop open or closing it." A personal need to believe in something—just as the necessity of a butcher's thumb—changes what's real. The butcher didn't think adding a few cents to the bill was dishonest but rather a necessity for keeping the doors of a marginal business open.

Sometimes being helpful involves living in the gray area of honesty. A client with advanced prostate cancer needed to decide between surgery and radiation. The oncologist was clear that waiting would have dire consequences since the cancer was aggressive and in the lymphatic ducts. Each procedure came with possible positive and negative outcomes, making a decision difficult. The procedures when weighed against each other appeared to be so equal my client felt unable to make a decision.[20] His wife assured him that whatever he chose she would support him but she thought surgery was a better option. His wife's opinion was what he needed to decide. He agreed to surgery. Later, she admitted to me that she was unsure which of the two procedures was better: "Most likely, they were equal, but not offering an opinion wouldn't have been helpful to him, and if the oncologist was correct, waiting until he could make a choice would have reduced the survival rate for either procedure." Honesty in this and many other instances can be an overrated virtue when compared with the needs of a loved one coping with cancer.

Suggestions

19. Being helpful may involve living in the gray area of honesty.
20. Your primary goal is to be supportive, not to assume the role of a judge.

BUILD TRUST EARLY

Establish trust well in advance of when you need it. The first part of a cancer journey might be routine, such as doing minor things you promised or bringing food items to the house when you said you would. As the trip continues, trust will become critical when your loved one depends on your counsel or feedback for crucial decisions. Trust involves the willingness of your loved one to expose her vulnerability and rarely happens through one interaction. The development of trust is a cumulative process with no specific number of interactions leading to it. Your loved one will be sending you two messages with each "trust trial." The first is *I'm sharing something that exposes my vulnerability. I trust you won't exploit it.* The second part of the message is *Your response will determine whether I will go further in trusting you.*

The more often you can provide evidence you are trustworthy, the quicker a trusting relationship will develop. Another factor affecting the development of trust is the importance of what transpires. The greater the "importance" load, the quicker you will establish trust. For example, a friend tells you his diagnosis in confidence and says, "Please don't tell anyone until you ask me if it's okay." He's trusting you not to reveal critical information. It's different than asking you to pick him up at a particular time. Being ten minutes late for the pickup can be annoying, but divulging the diagnosis can be as devastating to your relationship as it was for a man who feared discrimination if his supervisor knew about his cancer. A friend, who worked at the same company, promised not to tell anyone about the diagnosis. He didn't question his promise until witnessing the supervisor criticizing his friend for not moving fast enough. He faced a terrible dilemma: keep his promise and watch the supervisor chastise his friend or break his promise and confide in the supervisor, thereby making his friend's life easier but risking losing trust. After much soul-searching, he decided that even though he had promised his friend not to reveal the diagnosis, he couldn't stand by and watch the supervisor's abusive treatment. Out of compassion, he chose to tell the supervisor. It was the wrong decision. Once the supervisor knew why the man was moving slower, he apologized and the criticism stopped. The man was furious with his friend for betraying his trust. He had decided that under no circumstances would he reveal the diagnosis to the supervisor. Their history, unknown to his friend, involved the supervisor's taking advantage of employees' vulnerability. Although the supervisor's criticism stopped, he knew it was temporary and within weeks the abuse would continue. As the man's cancer progressed, he refused to accept help from his lifelong friend, who, he believed, had shown himself to be untrustworthy. Trust is a delicate relationship. Guard it as if it were a newly hatched chick.

You can also establish trust by listening nonjudgmentally. When I was a hospice volunteer, patients shared heartrending experiences with me. I realized their revelations had less to do with who I was and more to do with their need to establish trust with someone who would be present as they died. Your loved one may not be in jeopardy of dying, but he will still need to establish trust for the journey he's about to take. It becomes easier to approach difficult topics after trust had been established. An example is what a caregiver faced with a husband who had pancreatic cancer. She was a nurse and understood what he would be experiencing. She was supportive from the time of the diagnosis, yet honest with him about how his life would change. She explained the plans they made for their retirement would not happen, but she didn't dwell on the terminal nature of his illness. A more difficult conversation involved treatment decisions necessary as his illness progressed. She knew he would need to decide whether to continue a life-prolonging chemotherapy or allow the disease to progress. The trust she established throughout their two-year journey enabled him to listen and accept her recommendations.

Suggestions

21. Establish trust well in advance of when you need it.
22. The development of trust is cumulative. Each trustworthy action moves it forward.
23. Trust is difficult if not impossible to regain after you lose it.
24. Develop trust by doing what you say you will do, listening compassionately without judging, witnessing your loved one's pain without withdrawing, and skillfully balancing honesty with support.

SEND GOOD THOUGHTS

I heard from many people that the "good thoughts" they receive from friends and family are important. Many don't believe they will affect the cancer, but they make them feel better knowing someone cares. Others look at good thoughts as having a direct relationship to the outcome of their cancer. These positive thoughts, according to some mind-body advocates, can help with the healing process.[21] Regardless of what you believe, a bond is created when you tell people you have good thoughts about them. "My thoughts are with you," or "I'm praying for you," or "My heart is with you" conveys a partnership in something painful or dreadful.

Good thoughts can originate from religious convictions or secular beliefs. A religious person living with cancer took comfort from daily prayers offered in her name by friends in different parts of the country. She was uplifted when she joined them in long-distance prayer sessions. According to her, at noon, she stopped whatever she was doing and in prayer communed with friends and family throughout the country. It was the highlight of every day. Good thoughts emanating from secular beliefs can also create bonds. Friends of a patient who had no religious convictions formed a "good thoughts" group. Every day at a specific time, they collectively sent their thoughts telepathically to counteract the cancer. The woman was moved by their efforts, even as a research scientist, but she didn't think the practice would affect the cancer. Her motto in life was if it's not feelable, smellable, or seeable, it doesn't exist. What touched her was that her friends thought enough about her well-being that they would take five minutes every day to send good thoughts for her recovery.

Even though your friend may not share your religious beliefs, sending good thoughts or offering prayers is comforting. Many people experience loneliness at the start of their journey whether they live in a fourth-floor walk-up in the worst part of town or reside in the most exclusive suburb of San Francisco. People can experience isolation living in a large extended family or alone in an unfriendly city. I often receive emails from people offering prayers for my continued health since I write about living with prostate cancer. Most come from people whose religious convictions I don't share, but their concern always moves me. The purpose of offering good thoughts or prayers is not to share compatible religious views or proselytize but rather to do something to emphasize the bond between you and your friend.

If it's important to your faith for you pray for a complete recovery, do so. But statistics and logic indicate you shouldn't limit prayers to a complete cure. Almost fifteen million people in the United States live with cancer.[22] Of those, more than one and a half million will die every year despite many of these people having strong religious convictions.[23] Instead of offering only prayers for a cure, include areas necessary for end-of-life preparation, such as completing unfinished business, forgiving others, and asking for forgiveness from people wronged and thanking those who made life meaningful. By definition, a miracle is something occurring with limited frequency and against all odds. There is nothing wrong with hoping for a miracle, but you'll be more helpful to your friend by focusing on praying for manageable, incremental goals.

Suggestions

25. Sending good thoughts says to a person with cancer you care. It establishes a bond.
26. Good thoughts can be religious or secular.
27. Don't limit good thoughts to a cure.

HELP THE PERSON IN EMOTIONAL SHOCK TO FUNCTION

Often the term "shock" is used to describe changes in a person's behavior because of a traumatic physical event. Medical personnel go on high alert when any of nine physiological symptoms of physical shock occur.[24] But what should be done about emotional shock, the kind that happens when a person realizes his life is about to change in frightening ways? Rarely are efforts as intensive to stabilize a person in emotional shock as they are with physical shock. Many people who are still in shock after hearing a cancer diagnosis are required to make urgent choices, which include treatment options, who should be told about the diagnosis, what prior decisions should be reevaluated, and planning for a cancer-filled or shortened future.

A client of mine faced many of these issues following a leukemia diagnosis. He had been decisive his entire life but couldn't decide between two treatment protocols for an aggressive form of leukemia, nor could he make decisions such as *Should I close the sale on the dream house my wife and I found? Should I cancel the cruise we planned for the past year? Should I tell my boss and, if I do, when?* The more he pondered what he would face, the more "Should I" questions bubbled up. He was fortunate his wife relieved much of the burden from his shocked brain by guiding him in treatment choices and events having significant financial consequences. She became responsible, with his consent, for all day-to-day decisions until his emotional shock receded.

The length of time a person remains in emotional shock is less related to the severity of the prognosis and more to how accepting he is of the disease. Emotional shock for the above client lasted two weeks. Emotional shock for another client with an easily treatable cancer was longer. He was a high-level executive responsible for the finances of a Fortune 500 company. His oncologist assured him his bladder cancer was curable, but he still couldn't act because of his fears. Not only was he unable to function at work, but when asked to make decisions about his treatment he responded with "I don't know." His oncologist, who was focusing only on treatment protocols, emphasized that the sooner he made a decision, the better would be the outcome. The oncologist couldn't understand why his patient didn't recognize the importance of a quick decision since he made significant business decisions daily. His wife knew what her husband was experiencing and made sure she was present during every subsequent conversation between her husband and the physician. When the doctor insisted that her husband decide on a treatment option before he left the office, his wife assured him they would decide in a few days. Her gentle support allowed her husband to recover some of his emotional equilibrium. He didn't return to his prediagnostic emotional state, nor was he able to function at work, but he did improve enough to select a treatment option.

About 25 percent of all cancer patients who are in emotional shock will experience depression.[25] I found that the calming (some would describe them as "dulling") effects drugs create are often dependent on their continual use. Current research indicates that the total reliance on drugs to combat depression may not be warranted.[26] For some patients, drugs can be effective in reducing the effects of depression, but with others, it may not be helpful in the long-term acceptance of the diagnosis. Rarely are antidepressants alone sufficient for treating the emotional shock of a cancer diagnosis. Counseling may help, but your attitude and presence may be the most important variables. You can be supportive by helping your loved one focus on the specific things required to treat the cancer, such as making appointments and changing diets. Depression has a greater chance of occurring when the prognosis is terminal[27] since few people, even those possessing a spiritual attitude, are prepared to die after receiving a terminal prognosis.

Suggestions

28. There is no specific amount of time emotional shock will last.
29. Emotional shock can lead to depression.
30. Don't rely on drugs to stop emotional shock; use supportive actions.
31. Reduce the number of nonmedical decisions, delay medical decisions when possible, and assist your loved one to understand the consequences of each choice.

ACCEPT AND SUPPORT TREATMENT DECISIONS

Living with cancer involves choices. Sometimes they seem endless. We can choose to undergo invasive procedures or refuse them. We can choose to think of ourselves as doomed or coping with cancer. We can lead our lives as deniers, adaptors, or accepters of the disease. We don't choose between something pleasant and something terrible. Most options are bad, but some less so than others. For me, my choices started thirteen years ago. The options for treating prostate cancer were limited to watchful waiting, external beam radiation, radioactive implant seeds, surgery, and hormone therapy.[28] My cancer was too aggressive for watchful waiting and with a Gleason score of 7 the use of radioactive seeds was ruled out by the radiologist. The only options left were surgery or external beam radiation. There was the possibility of incontinence or impotence with surgery. With radiation, rectal bleeding and months of pain might occur. Not quite the same as choosing between eating at McDonald's or a three-star Michelin restaurant.

Without any medical training and still in emotional shock, I had to make a decision affecting the quality and possibly the length of my life. What I knew came from medical journals, anecdotal stories told by men with prostate cancer, and unsubstantiated claims made on the Internet. People with other forms of cancer face similar difficult choices. My primary care physician suggested I contact a respected San Francisco oncologist. He was in a position to evaluate the cancer and recommend the best treatment protocol. I relaxed when entering his office, believing a knowledgeable professional would help me decide between radiation and surgery.

After looking over my medical records, he said, "Well, it's six of one, half a dozen of the other." I was unimpressed with folksy wisdom coming from a highly respected elder of a prestigious medical school. "With surgery, there is an 85 percent probability you'll survive at least five years. With external beam radiation, you have an 81 percent probability." He leaned back in his chair as if waiting for me to look relieved. I liked the 85 and the 81 percentage figures, even if only five-year survival data were available. My mind, however, was drawn to the percentage of failures. For those of us with a potentially deadly form of cancer, "six of one, half a dozen of another" is not a witty sophism. What we experience in looking at "nonsurvival" figures can be frightening. No matter how optimistic one is, getting past even small failure rates is difficult.

"With my cancer," I said, "which of the two failure groups do I have the greater probability of dropping into?" I could tell this wasn't the type of statistical question posed to him by patients. I assumed other patients' ques-

tions focused on chances of survival, not death. I persisted when he equivo-
cated in a series of vague answers. "So are you saying that if I die, I chose
the wrong treatment?" He was even less pleased with my question. "How
can I be expected to choose the better treatment when you are reluctant to
take a position?" He hesitated before uttering a favorite medical line, "It's
the patient's choice." I wondered where I would find a new oncologist.

Scenarios such as this occur daily, and the odds are your loved one
found herself in one. "Choices" are often presented to patients as empow-
ering. If I studied medicine or approached the topic as an objective scientist,
choosing between the two options would have been easier. But this was
my life, and with only a small amount of medical knowledge, I didn't feel
empowered choosing between two procedures I didn't understand, with
very different side effects. Treatment choices are more ominous when
the cancer is uncontrollable. They can range from aggressive intervention
with severe side effects to refraining from treatment other than palliative
care (pain control). The choice is often between extending one's life with
unpleasant side effects or a shorter life with only palliative care but fewer
side effects. Your loved one's most significant decision may be choosing
or rejecting life-extending treatment. Don't offer an opinion on what you
would do in a similar position unless she asks. Support her decision even
if you disagree, but be comfortable in asking for clarification if she rejects
life-extending treatment.

Seven years after my diagnosis I was a guest of the South Korean
government for the opening of its Proton Beam Therapy Center. Proton
beam therapy is a more precise form of radiation.[29] I was invited because
of my publications on the health crisis in the United States and experience
as someone living with prostate cancer. In the morning, there would be an
official ceremony at the facility, followed by informational sessions with the
medical staff for the remainder of the day. Discussions of treatment options
brought back memories of my decision to have surgery rather than radiation. I learned from the South Korean medical staff that my question to the
oncologist in San Francisco was still unanswered. Where is the solid data
people with cancer need to make an "informed decision" about their treatment? The questions I posed thirteen years ago to the oncologist and seven
years ago to the South Korean medical staff still can't be definitively answered today. One often hears the mantra that consumers need to be proac-
tive and involved in the medical decisions affecting their lives. I agree, but
solid evidence, not personal convictions, should be the basis for decisions.

I was involved in a "patient's choice" situation a number of years ago,
when I was doing stuttering therapy. A client was adamant about going

through "rebirthing" therapy as a way of experiencing the moment when he began stuttering. I didn't say, "Well, if that's your choice, fine" or "Six of one, half a dozen of the other." I told him the therapy was ludicrous. I would like to think research drives treatment, but I don't think it always does. If it did, then more comparative studies looking at longevity and quality of life would be done. What I find tragic today is that most men facing treatment for prostate cancer are as confused as I was thirteen years ago. Asking patients—regardless of the type of cancer—to choose an intervention affecting the quality and length of their lives is often a cop-out for the medical community. Patient involvement doesn't negate physician responsibility in the decision.

Thirteen years have passed since I decided on surgery rather than radiation. Did I make the right choice? I don't know and never will. If my choice leads to a long period of cancer control, would my life span be even longer with the rejected treatment? If the surgery failed, would radiation have resulted in a better outcome? These unanswered questions create anxiety, which often increases before scheduled checkups or when something innocuous, but suspicious, occurs. I become anxious when I experience bone pain. For someone with breast cancer, a normal calcification lump in her breast tissue causes concern.

We often don't understand why our loved one made a poor decision, as was the case for a man who selected radiation rather than a combination of surgery and radiation for his Stage IV esophageal cancer. He made the choice knowing the side effects of both radiation and surgery. His friend tried to convince him to undergo both since the combination results in a better survival statistic than radiation alone.[30] Regardless of what he chose, the three-year survival rate was less than 30 percent and the five-year survival was an even more dismal 5 percent.[31] What his friend didn't know was that he had ignored the relevancy of survival statistics in making a decision. The most debilitating side effects of radiation wouldn't happen for months, giving him time to improve his relationship with his estranged daughter.[32] The price he would pay for radiation would be skin irritation, loss of appetite, fatigue, stomach problems, and pain while swallowing. Surgery would mean the immediate loss of his voice with the removal of his larynx, limiting his communication to writing.[33]

Simple criteria are rarely the basis for treatment choices, as illustrated in the above example. Your friend may be wrestling with many variables, such as *Which treatment produces the least aversive side effects? What will the different treatments cost? How long will the treatment last? What will the effects of each treatment be on lifestyle? How will each choice affect the quality of life? Which procedure will offer the best chance of survival?* Your friend may share some of these issues with you, but others will remain a mystery. Don't be afraid to ask factual questions about the selection. Ask why he's still choosing something inferior if you believe he made the wrong choice.

The decision to refuse or stop life-prolonging therapy is complicated. What's difficult for friends and loved ones to accept is why someone would choose to stop a life-extending intervention. *Shouldn't one want to live as long as possible?* Many people believe the extension of life, regardless of the physical cost, is worth the pain. It's a belief found in both Eastern and Western societies. Until recently, the culture of Taiwan made it almost obligatory for adult children to do whatever was necessary to extend their parent's life regardless of the cost to them and pain to their parents.[34] A woman in her eighties living in San Francisco had a very different view. She decided to enter hospice rather than allow her son and daughter-in-law to care for her. Her ideas about the quality of life involved the ability to think, something her glioblastoma was taking away. She could have lived longer without any pain by accepting the recommended intervention, but visions of what her life would become as her cognitive abilities dwindled became the basis of her decision. Your loved one's decision to stop all life-extending procedures is neither one-dimensional nor easy to make. Assume your loved one took everything into consideration before making such a momentous choice. All people should have the right to determine when they will die. In Chapter 7, the right to die, along with end-of-life topics will be covered.

Suggestions

32. Support difficult choices even if you disagree.
33. Ask for an explanation if you don't understand why your loved one made a decision with which you disagree.
34. A choice to end life-extending treatment is not a reflection on you.

3

A LIFE OF UNCERTAINTY

Someone asked me what living with cancer for thirteen years is like, never knowing whether the disease will remain under control. I said, "It's like being hurled into a classic 1950s horror movie where you know terrible things will happen but you don't know when they will occur." Many people treated for cancer, as I have, conjure up reoccurring thoughts during those quiet moments when the mind entertains what you've tried to repress all day. *When will it come back? Will it get more severe? When will I lose those things I love?* These questions and others inject anxiety into the most insignificant events. Many other expressions of concern are misinterpreted, such as the gratitude we express for even your smallest efforts, our lack of gratitude for what you have sacrificed, and our attempts to tamp down anxiety before routine medical visits. As we struggle to keep our fears in check other behaviors are misinterpreted such as craving simplicity, the desire for control, the need for stability, and what we interpret as "dignified treatment."

WHEN YOU BECOME COLLATERAL DAMAGE

Cancer is a community event bringing people along the journey whether or not they want to come. We interact with a stranger and wonder why she's so distant, not knowing she is struggling with the effects of a recent chemotherapy session. A salesperson ignores your question about a dress's material, and you interpret her nonresponse as hostile since you don't know how the recurrence of her cancer is disrupting her life. A good friend will no longer accept invitations to social events because of pain, and not knowing that she has cancer leaves you believing you did something wrong. I didn't realize the impact my prostate cancer would have on friends and family and even people who were casual acquaintances or strangers. The journey I and others with cancer are on produces collateral damage through our unskillful words and behaviors. When you don't understand why your loved one said something shocking to you or others or did something un-expected, assume the cancer generated it.

The course of cancer's development and treatment is not stable.[1] If it were, we could predict outcomes. Think of your loved one as trying to bal-ance on an exercise platform, a device physical therapists use to strengthen core muscles. Efforts to maintain balance must be continuous since remain-ing in one position without falling is impossible. In many ways, the balance board is analogous to living with cancer. Your loved one may be trying to balance acceptance of how the disease is limiting his life with resistance to the changes cancer creates. Even when assured a person is cancer free, the thought reoccurs: "But what if a few cancer cells remain?"

Suggestions

1. Treat cancer as a community event, not something owned by your loved one.
2. Much of what your loved one is feeling may be unshared.
3. Plan for instability rather than a predictable life.

HOW SIDE EFFECTS WILL CHANGE YOUR LOVED ONE'S LIFE

The world of side effects is unsettling, even if you know they are com-ing. I'm sure sometime in the future we will view contemporary methods of treating cancer as barbarous approaches to eliminating the disease. The purpose of all traditional protocols regardless of the treatment is to do one of three things: remove cancerous tissue, kill cells, or contain the cancer.[2] If you believe the commercials eliciting donations for research, we are close to defeating cancer, but until it happens, most treatments result in psycho-logical and physical side effects. Many people confine their thinking of side effects to those things that may or may not occur after treatment. This view disregards the distinctions between known side effects and side effects still unknown—a problem for all new treatments.

Known short-term and long-term side effects. Exhaustion is the most com-mon short-term side effect of cancer treatments. Forty percent of cancer patients report a loss of energy differing from the normal "tiredness" everyone experiences.[3] As cancer cells multiply, their growth robs nutrients from normal cells, resulting in a loss of energy.[4] The loss of energy is not only due to the growth of the cancer cells but can also occur from treatment effects. Up to 90 percent of patients treated with radiation and up to 80 percent of those treated with chemotherapy experience fatigue that continues for months and even years after the completion of treatments.[5] The psychological turmoil a person experiences also contributes to the loss of energy.[6] It can come from fearing a recurrence; the daily physical problems created by the cancer; treatment; and interactions with family, friends, and professionals.

A patient with liver cancer I served in hospice experienced wide swings in his energy level and presence of pain. Some days we walked on a beach in San Francisco for hours until I insisted we return because I was too tired to continue. On other days, he didn't have enough energy to use the bathroom. It was difficult for me to determine whether the growing tumor or coming to terms with the end of his life caused the exhaustion. The distinction between the two was less relevant than recognizing when it was occurring. You may be tempted to cajole a loved one to "get out of the house" or do something active rather than sit in front of a TV. Accept his claim of being too tired to move. "Willing" more energy is not effective, and neither is providing rewards for actions you think will be helpful ("If you walk to the end of the block, we can stop at the café before we come back").

My hormone treatments produce at least three side effects. The first is some discomfort at the injection site, followed by a strange sensation as the hormones begin shutting down testosterone production. A week later, I start menopause-like effects, except more intense, and coast along with the gradual reduction of side effects until the next three-month injection, when it starts again. I have been receiving the injections for the past thirteen years and still don't experience consistent physical reactions other than reduced energy. Assume the direct effects of treatment, its side effects, or contemplated future side effects are exhausting. Reduce the number of social events you are planning as a precaution or plan ones you believe will be doable for your loved one. She should not view the reduction of social events as exclusion from your life or the life of friends and family.

For many people, even "wonder drugs" can be a crap shoot when it comes to side effects. Take for example the drug Femara (letrozole), whose manufacturer claims halves the risk of cancer reoccurring or spreading from one breast to the other.[7] Side effects according to the manufacturer include hot flashes, hair loss, joint/bone/muscle pain, tiredness, unusual sweating or night sweats, nausea, diarrhea, dizziness, trouble sleeping, drowsiness, weight gain, weakness, flushing (warmth, redness, or tingly feeling), headache, constipation, pain in hands spreading to arms, and numbness/tingling/weakness/stiffness in hands or fingers or wrists, forearms, or shoulders.[8] Will every patient develop all these side effects? No, but the number and severity of them are indeterminate. What would you do if you were faced with deciding whether to use letrozole? You can take it to reduce the possibility of cancer spreading to your other breast, but the decision involves accepting the possibility of experiencing one or more of eighteen different side effects. Those of us living with cancer must balance the extension of life against the possibility of developing other problems. Sometimes those choices involve the selection of protocols and at other times, it's about deciding whether to take a drug.

Unknown future side effects. Future side effects of new medicines are unknown. A recent preliminary study linked the use of androgen deprivation therapy (ADT) in the treatment of prostate cancer with an increased risk of contracting Alzheimer's disease.[9] The article was of interest to me since I have been on ADT for the past thirteen years. Although the study was small (16,888 men with prostate cancer), the implications for my future are disturbing. The probability of a male developing Alzheimer's ranges between 6 and 9 percent, depending on which prevention factors are present.[10] After thirteen years on ADT, I now have a 12 to 18 percent probability of developing Alzheimer's. Nobody imagined Alzheimer's could be a side effect of this life-saving treatment when I began ADT. The uncertainty of the long-term side effects of cancer-fighting drugs can weigh on your loved one's mind. Not only is she balancing the life-saving effects of a drug against known side effects but also against unpredictable ones such as those that occurred with estrogen replacement therapy for women and now ADT for men.[11]

Side effects also can change a predicable response from someone living with cancer to an unexplainable lapse in compassion or judgment. A patient with lung cancer was so overwhelmed by his difficulty in breathing that he couldn't respond compassionately when a friend told him about the death of a relative. The friend was shocked since my patient always asked about his relative's health. His friend didn't realize he no longer had the emotional strength to offer condolences. Your loved one will vacillate between attentiveness to your needs and his emotions. The uncertainty of the future can overload his ability to be caring and compassionate.

Suggestions

4. Expect exhaustion from the effects of cancer and its treatment and side effects.

5. Accept the presence of treatment side effects ranging from mild to severe, none to many, those expected, and those not expected.
6. Reduce the number of scheduled social events.

THE MEANING OF GRATITUDE AND ITS ABSENCE

Gratitude is a strange animal. Both its absence and its presence in people living with cancer are often misunderstood. A lack of appreciation may indicate a reluctance that your loved one has in moving from independence to dependence. A retired educator in a San Francisco hospice facility refused help, sometimes risking injury because his cancer made physical movements more difficult. A compassionate staff person tried to assist him when he rose from bed. He not only refused her efforts but yelled at her. Accepting help meant he was dying, something he couldn't accept, even though he was in hospice and had signed a document acknowledging he had less than six months to live. Once, after he had screamed at the attendant, she said, "I know you don't want my help now, but I want you to know that I'll be here when you can accept it." For two weeks, he refused offers of help, causing himself needless pain. Staff members expected a painful injury if he didn't recognize the changes in his physical ability. Negative reactions from loved ones for your efforts are rarely about you. Unskillful words and actions are more often statements about how your loved one's life has been affected by cancer rather than anything you did wrong.

The flip side of ingratitude is excessive gratitude. Gratitude from someone living with cancer may be the acknowledgment of vulnerability and dependency. He is saying, "I can't do this anymore by myself." On one visit to the gentleman who refused help from the staff person, we discussed an interesting but irrelevant academic topic since both of us were retired university professors. For forty-five minutes he was again a respected researcher with an impeccable reputation as a scholar. His nurturing memories stopped when he realized his urinal was full. He asked me to empty the container, and with that request, his visions of independence and respect vanished. He was someone who could no longer do something as simple as taking care of personal hygiene.

He spent the next ten minutes thanking me when I returned from the bathroom. I thought the gratitude he expressed was out of proportion to what I had done, and I made the mistake of saying "It was nothing." In my mind, what I did was routine, a task I did for countless other patients.

For him, having to ask a full university professor to empty a urinal was humiliating and an undeniable signal he no longer could care for himself. We accept thank-yous as a matter of courtesy. In response we often say something such as "It isn't a problem" or "Don't worry about it; it's nothing." Don't minimize expressions of gratitude from someone living with cancer. Saying thank you for my patient was an expression of deep gratitude and an acknowledgment of his declining condition.

Gratitude can also be expressed as a reaction to fearing abandonment. When I was a hospice volunteer, I would take my patients for drives along the Pacific Coast Highway. The experience for most of them was calming since the drive from San Francisco to Bean Hollow State Park is one of the most beautiful sections of California State Route 1. I was troubled when one patient began crying as we drove. I asked whether there was anything he wanted to discuss. He said, "I'm afraid I'll keep living. Everyone has been wonderful to me, but how long can you do that? I'm afraid I'll outlive your compassion." His fear of being abandoned resulted in expressing deep gratitude for the most minor of services provided to him by staff. Listening to his thanks for someone dishing out a bowl of chocolate ice cream, one would think the person had just saved his life. Your loved one may contemplate an unexpected or unwelcomed life and wonder how long you will stay at his side as the disease tests your limits of compassion. It was a feeling expressed by a client whose husband went from "somewhat caring," according to her, prior to the cancer, to "excessively appreciative" as his cancer grew. People living with cancer who haven't experienced compassion over an extended period may find it frightening or a sign you will abandon her when the compassion well runs dry. The belief can result in heartfelt expressions of gratitude for minor actions.

Suggestions

7. Graciously accept gratitude as the expression of vulnerability.
8. Don't take personally a lack of recognition for your efforts.
9. Treat a lack of gratitude as a signal it's time to discuss resistance to increased dependence.

BE SUPPORTIVE AS EXAMINATION APPOINTMENTS APPROACH

For the past thirteen years, I have had a PSA test every three months. The examination becomes an event where the PSA number shapes my attitude toward life until the next examination. If it is below a threshold point, I can momentarily stop hormone therapy. If it is above the threshold, therapy and its side effects continue. If it is significantly above the threshold, the growing cancer requires a more invasive and debilitating intervention. Every three months I experience the medical version of the TV show *Let's Make a Deal.* After a contestant chooses one of three doors, Monty Hall opens the selection and reveals a prize ranging from a new car to a goat. Every three months I wait to hear whether I'm the owner of a new Cadillac or stuck with an unruly animal.

Most physicians suggest regular checkups even if cancer symptoms aren't present. In my conversations with people living with cancer, most of them are anxious as the examination date approaches. Even when their cancer is said to be "cured" or "in remission," they believe replication will occur if only one microscopic cell survived. The uncertainty of their status affects relationships with loved ones and friends, as mine does with my wife. She always knows a blood test is imminent by my behavior, which she kindly describes as "less than rational." The uncertainty of the blood test plays havoc with my emotions, as it does with most people's who go for regular checkups. Few people are calm as the date approaches. You can reduce the stress of an appointment by taking on your loved one's responsibilities such as grocery shopping or paying bills. Don't discuss confrontative issues until after his appointment since stress compromises the ability to cope with cancer.[12] If you can eliminate even a small amount of stress before the appointment, you'll give your loved one a better opportunity to handle the checkup's outcome.

Suggestions

10. Take on additional responsibilities as the appointment date nears.
11. Be supportive of what your loved one is experiencing rather than exhibiting unbridled optimism regarding the checkup's outcome.

HELP CREATE SIMPLICITY, STABILITY, AND CONTROL

In our high-tech society, simplicity isn't a cherished goal. We love to make everything complicated, from cell phones to relationships. Do the reverse to help your loved one—simplify. A Greek philosopher said, "I threw my cup away when I saw a child drinking from his hands at the trough."[13] There is a virtue in simplicity. It can take the form of decluttering your home, reducing the number of activities, or anything making life less complicated. Often, the unintended consequence of simplicity is increased structure and control, two important elements for introducing stability into your loved one's life. We often misunderstand the need for stability. Your loved one may insist certain things never change, such as when you serve dinner or how often you shop for groceries. You may grumble *What is the difference if dinner is at 6:00 p.m. or 6:15 p.m.? Why does a check for $20 need to be deposited today rather than tomorrow?* Assume the time he wants something to happen doesn't matter; his uncompromising nature is an attempt to retain structure in a changing world. Allow him, as much as possible, to determine when and how things should occur. From structure comes stability—something sought by people with progressive diseases.[14]

I witnessed the need for stability when my mother visited me in San Francisco many years ago. I was cancer free, had few concerns about longevity, and saw my mother three to four times a year. I became concerned when I came home and couldn't find her. The back of our house abuts a steep incline leading to a forested area. My concern turned to panic when I saw the open deck gate leading to the forest. My mother was in her early seventies and becoming confused when situations or discussions were anything other than linear. I raced down the stairs expecting the worst and saw my mother emerging from a stand of trees carrying a handful of leaves and twigs, smiling as if she had solved a complex puzzle.

"Mom, what are you doing?" I said, relieved.

"Straightening out the forest." When she saw my bewildered expression, she said, "From inside the house, it looked so messy. I thought it would be nice to clean it up a little."

"But, Mom," I said, "it's a forest."

She stared at me as if I didn't understand why this simple act was important. Now, twenty years after her death, I realize my mother's need to keep things neat and organized was her way of dealing with what I suspect was early dementia. For me, someone living with cancer, "straightening out the forest" became important. My need for structure takes the form of paying all incoming bills on a certain date, clearing off my desk before I begin writing, and other behaviors I'm sure people believe are odd. I often think back to my mother's efforts at tidying up the forest. I now realize she used structure to give stability to her changing condition. Those of us with active cancer have similar needs for structure. We experience changes caused by the disease, its treatment, or the anticipation of either one. The more unstable our health, the more important structure and stability become.[15] Even people who are "cured" look back and wonder whether the cancer will return. For those of us with lingering doubts about our survivability, structure enables us to hold on to what is familiar. "Straightening out the forest" for my mother was another way of making the ground less shaky, her attempt to grasp at stability in a dissolving world.

The need for stability is greater when cancer is virulent since the world is changing at a frightening pace. Loved ones with walking problems know they will soon need a wheelchair. Those who require oxygen anticipate increased flow settings. Loved ones experiencing pain prepare for higher morphine dosages. A client with lung cancer once said to me, "Every day I feel as if I'm on a ship in a storm." His life had been quite stable before the cancer; now everything was in turmoil. "When I steady myself for the back and forth roll," he said, "a wave hits on the side, and I'm struggling again to balance." Imagine for a moment that you have little control over your life. The causes may be an abusive boss, an unreliable car, or the constant traffic on your street keeping you awake. To stop the annoyances, you can take another job, find a new apartment, or use public transportation. But what if none of these choices results in acceptable consequences? If you quit work, you might not find another job. If you give up your apartment, you might become homeless. If you can't afford to repair or replace your car and public transportation isn't available, you are stuck in your neighborhood. A lack of control would, at the least, make you disagreeable. This is the situation many people with cancer experience either with the progression of the illness or its treatment.

Early in my cancer treatment, I wanted to exercise following a hormone injection, but I had only enough energy to change my pajamas. After thirteen years of experiencing the injection effects more than thirty times, you'd think I would plan on being listless for three to four days. The experience should have instructed me about what to anticipate, but it hasn't. My hope, *this time will be different*, ignores years of history. I still have little control over how I will feel after an injection. I still hope I'll be fine, but I'm amazed when I'm not. The period following treatment might be the only time your loved one experiences a lack of control, but for other people, such as a friend who lived with a rare blood leukemia, instability was always present. He thought of himself as a rag doll whose body and mind were manipulated by treatments keeping him alive. His control diminished as the cancer became more virulent. "It's as if I'm in prison," he said. "The only thing I can control is my bladder, and even that's changing." Without control, stability becomes more of a memory than a daily experience. Predictability also suffers as stability dissolves. You can do many simple things to add predictability to your loved one's life. For example, don't change what you promise to do. Ten minutes late may be inconsequential for you, but for a person living with cancer, having to wait may be another check in the "no predictability" column.

Disorganization also causes instability. Think about your loved one's emotional and cognitive ability as a twelve-inch pie. The daily necessities of living consume a large part of it. The remainder is used to address the physical and emotional aspects of living with cancer. She may wish for a greater capacity to deal with life, but only a twelve-inch pie is available. The constant turmoil resulting from disorganization may limit her ability to deal with cancer. You can help her by reducing or eliminating disorganization. Offer to help in one area not requiring her assistance. The effects should be immediate, as it was for a person who was exhausted because of treatments. A client was despondent when bills went unpaid, past due notices came, and the credit card companies assessed penalties and threatened legal action. His friend offered to come to his house every Friday, look through the correspondence, and pay the bills. The effort took less than ten minutes each week and made her friend's life less stressful. Tackle another area of disorganization when you complete one.

Years ago I was preparing for a thirty-day trip to Japan, where I would be tracing the history of the Japanese bamboo flute (Shakuhachi) and studying with master teachers. We would be traveling throughout the country by train, and the only personal items we could bring were those we could carry in one small suitcase and hold in our hands. My decisions on what to take or leave behind would affect the quality of this trip of a lifetime. Too many items, and the weight would be burdensome. Not enough of the right ones, and I might be forced to neglect some basic needs. You'll be facing similar decisions, but with more significant consequences, as you begin a treatment journey with your loved one. Trying to do everything you and he did before his cancer is an attempt to hold on to a past life, resulting in neglecting your current one. The key to adapting to the new burdens of your loved one's life is to prioritize, as I did for my Japan trip. Start eliminating what's not important and focus only on what is.

Suggestions

12. Strive to simplify your and your loved one's life.
13. Accept behaviors that enhance your loved one's sense of stability and control.
14. Introduce predictability.
15. Help organize your loved one's life.
16. Prioritize what's important for the cancer journey; then act on it.

INSIST ON TREATMENT WITH DIGNITY

Dignified treatment can involve honorific titles, giving responsibility for decisions, not taking economic advantage of, accepting the legitimacy of feelings, or as was the case with my wife, appropriate behaviors by medical personnel when she had her stroke. Medical teams came into her hospital room from neurology and cardiology. The first time an attending physician did grand rounds he ignored us, speaking to his interns as if we were invisible. I decided to do two things during his next visit. The first was insisting that he sit next to my wife instead of hovering over her. In hospice, I learned that personal relationships between patients and staff members often parallel their physical distance. A physician standing over a patient in bed implies an inequity. Both people at eye level imply equality, not regarding roles, but what it means to be human. The second thing I insisted on was conversations acknowledging our presence. My wife and I were more than a "lesson" for interns; we were active participants in her treatment.

Dignity not only involves relationships but also accepting your loved one's ideas about what it means to *him*. A carpenter who worked in the construction industry had a simple philosophy: "There is no reason I should have anyone work on my house. If I can't do it myself, it shouldn't be done." With his cancer, almost every home maintenance issue required more strength than he was capable of mustering. He believed his wife violated his dignity by hiring a handyman to do routine repairs. She understood her error after her husband said it was depressing having someone else assume the role of "man of the house." Her compassionate hiring of a handyman was as undignified for her husband as was the decision made by the daughter of another patient. The daughter couldn't understand why her elderly mother objected to a professional male caregiver bathing her since cleanliness was important in her mother's life before the cancer. For the daughter, modesty had a much lower priority than being clean since an infection was more likely without bathing. She preferred to remain in soiled clothes rather than experience the humiliation of being washed by a male stranger. The daughter insisted that her mother allow the male caregiver to bathe her since she wasn't capable of doing it and the home care agency said a female caregiver wasn't available. Her mother complied, but her acceptance of the male caregiver created an irreparable gap between mother and daughter.

Your loved one may misinterpret helpful gestures as attacks on dignity. Basic cleanliness in the daughter's mind was more important than modesty. For her mother, who had been a well-respected and high-profile attorney for forty years, being bathed by a man was the worst indignity she could imagine. Don't assume the presence of a serious disease trumps beliefs of what your loved one considers dignified. What is practical and necessary to you may be undignified to your loved one. What's "dignified" is often a balance between values and needs. Don't assume your loved one's needs will outweigh what he views as dignified treatment as the cancer forces greater dependence. Always ask whether what you are proposing is acceptable.

Suggestions

17. Insist that your loved one is more than a "cancer patient" or a medical lesson.
18. Accept your loved one's designation of what's dignified.
19. Always ask whether what you think should occur is acceptable to her.

BALANCE INDEPENDENCE AND DEPENDENCE

Increased dependence can signal that the cancer is growing. The fears it generates may take the form of odd behaviors.[16] For example, a patient with bone cancer refused to use a walker, despite risking a debilitating fall. Accepting assistance in even the most limited form (e.g., using a walker) signaled that his life was changing in unacceptable ways. He was able to accept help only after realizing his progressive disability was not going to reverse. You'll be balancing independence with assistance as physical abilities change. Accepting your help may require your loved one to accept the limitations the disease imposes. If you assume he can handle a greater degree of independence than he is capable of, he may misinterpret your good intentions as a sign of not caring. Take your lead from him and don't be afraid to ask whether he needs help (e.g., "Would you like to clear the dishes or should I do it?") before you assume he needs help.

Independence and dependence aren't static. What your loved one refused today may be welcomed tomorrow. I learned about the importance of independence from hospice patients who experienced dramatic declines. They were dying, and even though their independence dwindled on a daily basis, doing whatever they were capable of without help was important. Your loved one, as my patients, may be moving from independence to dependence, from being in control to having less control. These transitions involve discomfort, sometimes even fear.[17] You can reduce anxiety by helping your loved one hold on a little less tightly to what is familiar.

Refusing to let go of dwindling abilities prevents loved ones from moving forward.[18] Assume many things in your loved one's "pre-illness" life will lose their permanence. Provide options (e.g., "Would you like to feed yourself or would you like me to hold the fork?") or ask direct questions (e.g., "Do you need help getting into bed?") as dependence increases. The adult son of a patient tried to anticipate his father's needs. He said to me, "To wait until he is in trouble would be disrespectful." What he didn't realize was that the constant anticipation had the reverse effect. The father interpreted his son's compassionate efforts as taking away from him the last visages of control. The transition between independence and dependence is similar to the Tibetan concept of the "Bardo," the psychological space between life and death.[19] The instability created by moving from independence to dependence distorts reality, as it did with my brother-in-law's belief that he didn't need a cane even though his brain tumor affected his ability to walk.

Suggestions

20. Ask your loved one whether she needs assistance before providing it.
21. Assume the balance between independence and assistance continually shifts.
22. It's better to be overly helpful than not helpful enough.
23. As independence declines, reinforce it, even if it involves inconsequential behaviors.
24. Help your loved one let go of parts of her identity that no longer exist.

LOOK FOR THE LOST EMOTIONS BEHIND GRIEF

The belief that substitutes for the loss of cherished activities aren't possible can lead to long-term grieving.[20] Those of us involved in serving people who are in emotional pain try to understand what's behind expressions of grief. The answers aren't as straightforward as many believe, as was the case with me because of cancer. I did solo wilderness fly-fishing throughout my adult life. It was the most enjoyable activity I ever did. I mourned its loss as if a close family member had died. When I understood that my grief wasn't about the loss of fishing, I searched for the emotion behind it. What did I experience standing in the middle of the McCloud River miles away from civilization? It wasn't the act of fishing or landing a trophy trout. I realized it was "serenity" I missed. My search for activities to re-create the lost emotion led me to craft and play wooden flutes. Did I find the same degree of serenity I had lost? Not quite, but playing a flute that I had made gave me a feeling similar to the one I had when I stood in the McCloud.

In our stratified society, we tend to analyze and subdivide everything. The same is true for grief. Specialty grief counselors exist for the dissolution of relationships, the death of a spouse, a sibling, a child, and pets. Each type of loss is thought to be unique and requiring a different specialist. But grief is grief, regardless of the type of loss generating it. In Chapter 8 we'll explore the nature of grief and ways of getting over it. For now, focus on not looking for a direct replacement for your loved one's loss; instead, search for anything to regenerate the lost emotion.

The length of time a loved one experiences grief depends on a simple choice: search for an exact replacement of the lost ability or activity or try to regenerate the associated emotion through a full range of activities or different goals. Choosing the first approach often leads to grief becoming a lifelong acquaintance, as it almost did for me. I was an avid runner, participating in marathons and one triathlon. I stopped when hip pain made even slow jogging difficult. What followed was a less than successful hip replacement because of a loss of bone density following years of ADT for my cancer. I compared what I had been capable of doing with what I was able to do after the hip replacement and found the difference depressing. If I focused on how much running ability I had lost, I still would be grieving. Instead, I decided to change my running goals. I no longer cared how fast or the number of miles I ran. Rather I tried re-creating the emotion I had before the hip pain. I found it on a crisp fall morning running alone on a country road in the North Carolina mountains. Granted, I ran slower than my wife did thirty-five years ago when she was eight months pregnant—but the joy returned. I still run slower than many people walk but I'm happy doing it.

Think about a favorite activity that is no longer possible, for example, a woman's husband loved wood sculpting. The activity might indicate a love of creativity. He also constructed furniture requiring precision measurements and cuts. When he could no longer do either, his wife tried involving him in activities requiring creativity and precision behaviors. She hoped that reorganizing the storage area in their home might trigger creativity and designing a precise pattern for a flower bed might tap into his love of precision. Don't assume "substitutions" will replace a lifelong activity, but even brushing against the lost emotion is better than mourning its absence. The goal of living with cancer is to adapt. To live as if cancer or its treatment is inconsequential may be fine for some, but for most of us, it's a formula for making life tedious.

Suggestions

25. Don't try to replace the lost ability or activity. Rather, help your loved one find activities to regenerate the emotions.
26. Grief doesn't have a timetable or steps taking you from despair to joy.
27. Help your loved one shift the focus from unobtainable goals to smaller achievable ones.

DON'T ASSUME YOUR LOVED ONE IS AWARE OF INTERPERSONAL PROBLEMS

Sometimes disease or pain reduces awareness of what we say and do. The side effects when I receive hormone injections are almost identical to menopause, except more severe.[21] At parties, I often joke that I am the only man in the room who understands what women in menopause experience. It took a while to realize my mood swings were not caused by someone's comments but rather by the hormones raging in my body. I still have a tendency to blame others for my emotional instability, although I have repeated this cycle for thirteen years following the injections. My awareness of changes in my personality or mood is harder to detect since the transition from the amicable Stan to the annoying one is gradual. The same phenomenon occurs with other people living with cancer.

Don't confront your loved one when her unskillful behaviors are occurring. The discussion will often set off defensive reactions. I never want to hear what an ass I become while the drugs are playing havoc with my body's chemistry. Wait until there's a calm before providing feedback in the form of facts and how your loved one's behavior makes you feel. For example, "Yesterday you yelled at me for not having dinner ready on time (facts). Your yelling made me feel you didn't appreciate what I do for you (feelings)." Contrast this approach and the emotions generated by the statement "How can you be so inconsiderate?" When I realized the hormones were causing mood swings that were affecting the relationship with my wife, we discussed strategies to use. We ruled out lengthy explanations by my wife because I probably wouldn't be listening and, if I were listening, I probably wouldn't accept them regardless of their validity. We agreed to use a code phrase as an alternative. *Stan, wouldn't you like to spend some time by yourself at the cabin?* I never become defensive when she says the phrase since I realize I've become intolerable.

Your loved one can look back on his unskillful words and say, "This is what I should have done," but by then relationships may have been damaged. The simplest and most effective way of dealing with a fiasco is for you to encourage him to apologize to the people he insulted. A best friend of a woman coping with the side effects of chemotherapy didn't understand the severity of her abdominal pains. The woman with cancer became furious at her friend over an inconsequential remark. The interaction was so hurtful to the friend that she stopped all contact and refused to accept an apology. Sometimes your loved one won't be able to make things right. I damaged personal and professional relationships that weren't reparable during my initial treatments. I took solace in knowing I tried to apologize even though my efforts were unsuccessful.

Suggestions

28. Don't confront your loved one when the unskillful words or behaviors are occurring. Do it when they cease.
29. Confine your feedback to facts and how you felt when you explain the effects of hurtful behaviors and words. Don't frame the discussion as "this is what you did wrong."
30. Use code phrases as a shortcut feedback approach.
31. Accept a loved one's apology for inappropriate words or behaviors without being judgmental.

THINKING IS NOT THE KEY TO HAPPINESS

At a workshop I led on change at a West Coast retreat center, one participant told me this was his tenth weeklong workshop in the past five years. "Why so many?" I asked. "I'm looking to find joy in my life." What I wanted to say was "Why not stop looking and do something?" I nodded instead as if I understood, but I didn't. Living with cancer can be a joyless state of being. You may be compelled to bring happiness into your loved one's life, but how to do that may be a mystery. There's an old story about a student who would sit meditating for long periods of time, waiting to be engulfed by enlightenment. A teacher, watching him for weeks, sat next to him and grabbed a piece of broken pottery. Without looking at the student or saying anything, he placed the shard in his lap and began rubbing it with a filthy cloth. After two hours of watching the old man, the student asked a question.

"What are you doing?" he said.

"Making a mirror."

"But how can you make a mirror by polishing a pot shard with a cloth?"

"How can you become enlightened by just sitting?"

I try to do three enjoyable activities every day: play my flute, carve wood, and write. Even when I do all three on a bad day, it may not compensate for what I experienced, but my mental state is better than if I did nothing positive. Reduce the impact of what's negative by helping your loved one experience something joyful every day. Search for simple things to bring joy into his life. Happiness doesn't require big gestures or deep thoughts. In the simplest of activities there is joy. Think about the cancer as a bully sitting on one end of a seesaw weighed down by negativity. To change the dynamics, you'll need to add weight (joy) to your loved one's side. Even though you may never be able to place enough weight on her side of the fulcrum to get her on the ground, you can get her closer. The same applies to cancer. Don't look to overcome it but rather strive to adapt.

There will be times when no matter what you do, there will be no joy. During a downward spiral the greater the grief, the more difficult depression will be to reverse. Counseling, when affordable, available, and acceptable to your loved one, can be helpful.[22] But if one of these necessary ingredients is missing, you may wonder what will work. Start with looking for something for which your loved one is passionate. The activity can be as simple as listening to her favorite music or walking on a level hiking path. Passion can introduce sufficient joy to reduce the effects of cancer to acceptable levels. I follow two important universal rules of change when helping people modify behaviors caused by chronic illness. The first is to maximize what's enjoyable and minimize what's unpleasant. The suggestion sounds as trite as the joke about a man who visits a physician. "Doctor it hurts when I do this," he says, raising his arm. "Then don't do that," the doctor responds. The maxim may be trite but rings true. Stop doing things causing pain or anxiety. The second universal rule is to make the change almost as easy as not changing. For example, if your wife loves walking but is afraid of tiring far from the house, walk only to the end of the block so she will be neither anxious nor exhausted. Other universal rules of change exist, but focus on these two and you should see a difference in her level of joy.[23]

Suggestions

32. Don't try to increase your loved one's happiness by talking or thinking.
33. Help your loved one find three positive things to do every day.
34. Rely on your loved one's passion for selecting positive activities.
35. Help your loved one stop doing negative things and replace them with positive ones.
36. Make change almost as easy as not changing.

4

THE NATURE OF LOSSES

There's an old Tibetan saying: "You can't have meat without the bone nor tea without the leaves." This view of life also applies to anything that gives us joy—grief is the price we pay for experiencing joy. Even if your loved one accepts the necessity of grief, it doesn't negate the anger he feels for having something taken away. The anger can be very intense; it distorts words and actions. Identities change when the losses are significant. With new identities comes the reordering of priorities. What was important before the cancer may now be insignificant and vice versa. When you don't recognize the changes, your expectations of what your loved one thinks, believes, and does become based on his precancer condition.

LOSSES ARE A PART OF LIFE

Many people who experience a loss react to life as if the music had stopped. We want life to remain stable or, even better, soar with pleasure. The misguided view regarding life's projectory appears in an old Zen story. A dejected student says to his Master, "I had a terrible meditation session." The teacher nods his head and responds, "It will pass." The next day the student again seeks out the teacher and says, "I had a great meditation session!" The Master nods his head and again says, "It will pass." Life for the Zen Master involved accepting a loss for what it is—an unavoidable part of living, something containing both pleasure and pain. Every one of us will experience joy and loss throughout our lives. One feature differentiating people living with cancer from each other is how we react to losses. The noted musician Wynton Marsalis said during a PBS interview that his grandmother's favorite expression was "life has a board for everyone's backside." It's a realistic view of what most people experience.

People who don't live with cancer often assess the magnitude of a loss from their perspective. For example, a husband who is a runner doesn't understand why his wife is so distraught about not being able to knit because of bone pain. After all, his reasoning goes, "It's not like she can't walk anymore. Now that would be a terrible." His wife's life centered around knitting. She did it weekly at a knitting club, while watching television, and in the car when her husband drove. Knitting was not just a casual activity; it was central to her social life and creativity. Her loss is far more devastating than being unable to walk. Any loss that a loved one maintains is substantial is by definition substantial.

I hear assertions that people diagnosed with cancer don't change. *He's no different now after receiving a cancer diagnosis than he was before the diagnosis.* Don't underestimate the powerful effect of a life-threatening diagnosis regardless of how "normal" we act. How we view ourselves—our identity—is based on many things: what we do, the roles we play, activities we enjoy, our affiliations, the values structuring our lives, and our abilities and relationships. These things together form our identity—something unique for every person. Eliminate one significant element and a person's identity changes.[1] Believing it doesn't would be like a waiter telling you the Eggs Benedict you received without the Hollandaise sauce is still Eggs Benedict.

People try to be supportive when losses occur by using "the glass is half full" point of view—*Yes, I know you can't jog anymore because of cancer, but don't forget what you're still capable of doing.* How convincing is the argument when the lost activity is a central feature of a person's life? Someone who nightly strolled with his wife and can no longer walk views his loss to be as significant as the cancer-free marathon runner who is devastated by the inability to compete due to a strained ligament. Cancer results in life-changing losses. Activities such as running, walking, writing, and knitting may disappear, but their memories remain, tormenting the person who can no longer do them. Ask anyone who experienced a significant loss what she thinks about "but look" propositions. It's a battle between the head and the heart: the head says relish what you're still capable of doing, but the heart mourns the loss.

Suggestions

1. Accept the changes in your loved one's personality because of a significant loss.
2. Don't use the "glass is half full" argument.

LOSING WHAT GIVES JOY

Each of us derives joy from different activities. A major source for me was teaching. I was a person who juggled multiple projects as a university professor before my sleep deprivation became acute. When someone asked what my profession was, I would respond, "Which day of the week?" My life changed as problems with my memory increased. I missed appointments and lost concentration when clients spoke about problems, my family thought I was ignoring their needs because I didn't care, and my students, well, let's say they were having doubts about my sanity. For months I lectured on automatic pilot, presenting material I knew so well. A coherent presentation was possible even when I had only a few hours of sleep. I had just finished a three-hour lecture following a sleepless night when my graduate assistant came into the office.

"Stan, can I talk to you about your lecture today?"

"Sure. What questions do you have?" I said as she closed the door behind her.

"I don't have any questions, but I need to tell you that . . ." She had difficulty continuing.

We had established a close student–mentor relationship where she was comfortable discussing both academic and personal problems with me. Whatever this was, I knew it was beyond the scope of previous conversations.

"Did I say anything factually wrong in my lecture?"

"No."

"Did I say something insensitive or insult anyone?"

"No."

"Then what?

"The lecture was fine." She paused before taking a deep breath. "But it was the one you gave last week."

"You mean I covered some of the same topics?"

"No. It was the same lecture, almost word for word." After a pause, she said, "Even the same jokes."

She went on to tell me the students were bewildered. It wasn't the first time my attempt to hide my memory loss had resulted in misconceptions at the University. After not sleeping for more than a few hours a night, I would stagger down the hallway in the morning, appearing to be intoxicated. Some outraged students even complained to the department chair, who knew of my sleep disorder but couldn't explain it to the students since I told him not to tell anyone. I decided to retire, not because I wanted to, but because my failing memory and perpetual exhaustion made it impossible to teach. For six months, between the time I informed the chair of my decision and the end of the semester, I asked myself how I could give up teaching. Teaching wasn't just something I did for thirty years; it was a significant part of my identity. Within six months, I was forced to give up a career and activities that gave me joy. I would face humiliation if I remained a teacher since I would no longer appear competent. I wouldn't provide my clients with the help they needed if I continued doing therapy. I might die if I didn't stop fly-fishing and canoeing alone in the wilderness.

Although my loss was not cancer related, its effects parallel losses resulting from cancer. There is no differentiation between types of grief or their significance when compared to each other. Grief is grief. The loss of memory caused by sleep deprivation spread through my life, affecting most aspects of my daily functioning. My life centered around academia, and I was being forced to give it up. Don't expect the loss to remain in only one area of your loved one's life as cancer takes away her favorite activities and skills. The tentacles of loss reach deep into your loved one's daily life.

Suggestion

3. Expect changes in your loved one's behaviors if the losses are significant.

ANGER

I was angry about how cancer was changing my life. It is a feeling I often heard from clients I counseled and coached. Most of us who experienced losses had "played by the rules," more or less, and because we had, the losses seemed unjustified. Many clients became angry believing they did nothing to deserve having a cherished activity taken away by cancer. The effects of the anger they experienced are analogous to a cup of liquid spilled on an unlevel table. No matter how quickly you try to clean it up, some of it will elude you, moving around on the tabletop and dropping to the floor. And as water spreads, so does the anger affecting parts of your loved one's life, his life unrelated to the loss.

The source of some anger is external. I assumed my colleagues at the University would commiserate with me when I told them I was retiring because of my memory problems. The less compassionate ones allowed their irritation to show since my retirement would result in a loss of financial support from the projects I headed. I couldn't understand why they weren't more concerned with my physical condition. *Didn't they realize what was happening to me? Why weren't they more understanding?* What I failed to realize was that my loss would also become their loss and their irritation was the flip side of my anger. The anger your loved one feels may be short-lived or long term, or internally or externally generated. Regardless of the form it takes, anger often distorts reality. While your loved one remains angry, it may be difficult to reason with him. There's an old Tibetan saying that "you can throw hot coals at the enemies but in so doing you'll burn your hands." Try to help your loved one dissipate his anger. Sometimes replacing anger with understanding makes it possible. I did that with the anger toward my colleagues when I realized my cancer would result in a significant disruption of their professional lives.

Suggestions

4. Expect your loved one's anger to spill into areas not related to his losses.
5. The anger expressed can be generated internally and through external reactions to the loss.
6. Expect anger to distort reality.
7. Don't marginalize your loved one's anger or take it personally.

DISTORTIONS

Losses can distort what a person living with cancer experiences.[2] The more consuming your loved one's grief, the more opaque her vision may become. Your loved one is not just going to a movie with you but going to a movie with you in pain. The perfectly prepared meal you spent hours making is no longer satisfying since his digestive system is impaired. It was a lovely walk you had with your wife, but she views it as an inadequate substitute for her daily run. Doors open if you view losses without anger, suspicion, and self-pity. My thoughts distorted efforts people made to help me such as my wife redirecting my driving when I made wrong turns. My adult son's and daughter's gentle reminders about important events made me feel like a child. My reluctance to accept help and rely instead on distortions had more to do with not accepting the loss than anything else. Our minds are tricky. Sometimes it's easier to hold on to misperceptions rather than to accept the loss.

Suggestion

8. Expect to see distortions.

DON'T FILL UP TIME

A common approach to compensate for losses is to fill a person's life with activities. People living with cancer often misunderstand this compassionate approach. One client said he was astounded by his wife's offer to buy him a puppy when he no longer could hike. "I hiked every weekend, sometimes for more than ten miles," he said. "How will a puppy replace that?" His wife's offer was genuine and heartfelt, but her husband perceived her suggestion as insensitive. Don't search for time "fillers" as the cancer or treatments strip away activities and abilities. Focus on why your husband enjoyed the activity he can no longer do. In the above example, the man's wife eventually understood the role of hiking in her husband's life. For him, hiking was not about exercise or the accomplishment of walking for ten miles. The activity provided him with a psychological space that allowed thoughts to settle. Together, they explored replacing the lost emotion, not the six hours that hiking occupied each week. Since his cancer was progressive and treatment effects were ongoing, they tried various options, until they rented a small boat and cruised the California Delta. The experience of cruising resulted in feelings similar to those he had while hiking. He and his wife focused on re-creating the emotion associated with hiking, not the replication of the activity.

Suggestion

9. Don't search for "time fillers." Rather, find activities appropriate to your loved one's new identity.

EXPECTATIONS FOLLOWING LOSSES

We act in line with expectations. We bite into an apple and expect it to be sweet rather than taste like vinegar. We say hello to someone and expect a greeting in return. We seek solace or a simple favor from a friend, and we expect him to respond as compassionately as he did in the past. From past behaviors come current and future expectations. Expectations should be modified when a significant loss occurs. The simple task your loved one performed before her loss now may be something either difficult to do or unimportant compared to what she is envisioning as her new life.

People living with cancer expect loved ones to understand how they changed because of a loss. My family was more compassionate than my university colleagues, but my behaviors still hurt them. A continual problem was forgetting birthdays and anniversaries even when I wrote them in my calendar because I forgot to review my commitments. On one occasion my daughter spent four hours preparing a gourmet dinner that I completely forgot about, remembering only when she called me at a friend's house as I was finishing dessert. Neither understanding nor compassion automatically translates into acceptance.[3] Losses often result in behaviors perceived as deliberately hurtful, as it did with my daughter. We tend to be oblivious to the effects of our behaviors when a significant loss consumes us. What we are certain of is that we've changed. You may have difficulty adjusting your expectations when losses change your loved one's personality. The "Stan" my wife knew for thirty years and my children for their entire lives was gone, yet expectations of me remained the same. I was a fixer of objects and people. Rarely did I hire a handyman to do anything around the house. Professionally, for thirty years I was involved in facilitating changes in behavior. I thought people's expectations of me should change since I knew I was a different person, but they didn't. *How can anyone expect me to be caring when I don't know how much longer I'll live? How can people expect me to remain my "happy self" when I can no longer do those things that gave me joy?*

Suggestions

10. Don't expect your loved one to act as he did before the loss of a significant ability or activity.
11. Base your expectations on your loved one's new identity, not on one that no longer exists.

ACCEPT REORDERING OF PRIORITIES

When a physician says you have a potentially fatal condition, your beliefs and values are shaken. What was important to your friend before the diagnosis may become irrelevant when he acknowledges that the possibility of dying soon is not theoretical.[4] Don't assume that what was important before the diagnosis is still important and, conversely, what was insignificant remains so. For example, distinctions between various coffees were important to a connoisseur before his cancer journey. He spent hours with fellow coffee lovers debating "important" distinctions such as the flavor and aroma of various countries' offerings. The discussions paralleled the chatter you hear when wine connoisseurs gather to rate obscure wines. *Is the Nicaragua*

Ocotal more buttery than the Sumatra Buah-Buahan? Does the India Tree-Dried Mallali Estate exhibit a more spicy finish than the Ethiopian Sidamo? He and his fellow coffee connoisseurs would spend hours every other weekend doing "cuppings" of exotic coffees. Nobody believed what they were doing had any importance other than to their palates. My client's interests changed following a lung cancer diagnosis. Hours spent sampling coffees lost its importance compared to end-of-life issues he faced and discussions with his family he knew were necessary. Although he shared his diagnosis with his coffee friends, they didn't understand why he no longer wished to participate in the cupping activity—something they had been doing for more than ten years. His friends' interpretation was that the cancer either depressed him or was affecting his ability to taste. Both explanations were incorrect. He reassessed what was important when he realized his life might be short. Spending eight hours every month sampling coffee became trivial compared with spending the time reengaging with relatives and old friends. What was viewed as something negative (e.g., giving up an important activity after the diagnosis) was in fact positive.

Friends and loved ones often don't understand how priorities held for a lifetime can change almost overnight with a cancer diagnosis.[5] There's an old story about a forgetful monk who couldn't remember at the end of the day whether what he did was virtuous. An older monk said to him, "For each thing you do, call it 'virtuous' or 'unskillful.' If it's virtuous, put a white pebble in your pocket. If it's unskillful, put a black one in it. When you come back to the monastery, sort the pebbles into two piles. If there are more whites than blacks, you had a good day." In many ways, those of us living with cancer go through life as did the forgetful monk, figuratively counting the number of white and black pebbles in our pockets. I count my pebbles at the end of each day and ask, "Did I do things today high on my priority list or did I ignore what is important and waste my time on lower priority items? I had a good day if I have more whites than blacks, more high-priority activities than lower ones.

Often in the face of adversity, we try to be supportive by identifying what will make a loved one feel better and then pushing it as a priority. A woman who followed world events before her diagnosis was no longer interested in how Middle Eastern countries are fighting terrorism. Outrage over events she couldn't control became unimportant in comparison to the preparation necessary for a lumpectomy followed by radiation. Her friends still tried to discuss world politics with her, not understanding the shift in her priorities. They thought, *This is something she was passionate about before the diagnosis, maybe we can use it to lift her spirits.* Context and passion are related. For example, the woman was interested in world politics when she believed she might be able to affect it (i.e., discussing the problem with others, financially contributing to a cause, getting involved, etc.). That's the context of her passion regarding world politics. Change the context—substitute a reduced life span for one appearing indefinite—and the passion may change. Instead of assuming priorities are unchanged or only minimally affected following a cancer diagnosis, become aware of your loved one's context.

Suggestions

12. Don't assume that what was important before the diagnosis is still important and vice versa.
13. Adjust your behaviors and expectations to the new context.

THE BIGGER PICTURE

At times we become consumed with specifics, ignoring the bigger picture. Your husband isn't staying on a pill schedule, so you talk about the importance of ingesting drugs when they are prescribed, going into detail about the consequences for being less than rigorous. Your wife doesn't want to do the exercises her physical therapist said were necessary for recovery following the mastectomy. Your response is to chastise her; unless she begins exercising, she'll delay her recovery. When she disregards your logical suggestions (e.g., you'll never get better by ignoring what you should be doing), you're baffled by her resistance. It may be time to explore the bigger picture when your loved one's decisions don't make sense. One elderly mother whose cancer was progressing refused to eat or drink. Her daughter's interpretation was that this was her mother's way of getting attention. It was a reasonable conclusion since her mother had been manipulative her entire life. The mother's conversation with her sister revealed another explanation: She believed it was time to die, and refusing to eat or drink was a conscious decision made to hasten her death. She wasn't trying to manipulate anyone. Not eating and drinking was a behavior acknowledging the end of life.

I believe it makes sense to assume your loved one's decisions are logical even though they may appear bizarre. For example, if your husband understands the importance of walking and chooses not to, angry words and threats will not be effective in changing his behaviors. He is choosing to become an invalid. While it may appear ridiculous to you, it might be the most rational choice for your husband if he weighed the importance and cost of both decisions and concluded that the rehab program would be too painful to justify the effort required. Ask the professionals responsible for the program to modify it, but be prepared for resistance. You may hear statements such as "It won't work if we make it easier." This type of response often comes from conscientious professionals who don't understand the principles of personal change.[6]

"Inappropriate" and "strange" are labels used when describing the behaviors of some people living with cancer. I often hear phrases such as "He never did that before the diagnosis" and "I don't understand why he's doing it now." Many of the behaviors loved ones cite as bizarre are often more "different" than "strange." A patient with bone cancer knew his life was limited. Even if treatment could control his cancer, things wouldn't be the same as they were before the diagnosis. His friends couldn't understand his decision to buy an expensive car since he would be able to drive it for only a few months. For my client, it was his last chance to own a new car—something he never could afford.

The stranger the behaviors, the more likely they result from hidden causes, often ones we identify as "last chances" or a "bucket list."[7] In the case of my client, many would say his "last chance" decision to buy a new car was justified. But how do you explain similar decisions by people with an active but treatable cancer, cancer in remission, or even cancer thought to be "cured"? The unpredictability of the disease can generate incomprehensible decisions. Not understanding the impact of a cancer diagnosis can lead to misunderstandings, as they did with a woman with a treatable skin cancer who visited so many foreign countries that her exhaustion affected her health. Friends couldn't understand why she did it. After all, what was the rush? In the woman's mind, the presence of a curable cancer highlighted her coming closer to dying: *Why not enjoy myself today when I don't know what tomorrow will bring?*

Did the above decisions make sense? Not if you try to understand them from the perspective of someone who isn't ill. Traveling alone with a serious condition seems foolish. Buying a new car when a person knows he will never use it is illogical. Along with cancer comes expectations of the future, ones we hope for and others we dread. We are members in a group of fourteen million people who live with cancer, and we know almost six hundred thousand of us, a little more than 4 percent, will die every year in the United States.[8] Why should we expect not to be in this category?[9] The uncertainty of life with cancer can lead to "bizarre" behaviors in both the "surviving" and "terminal" groups.

Never label behaviors as "bizarre" or "out of character" until you understand your loved one's reasoning. Think of these behaviors as having two different levels of meaning: what is obvious (e.g., wasting money on a car he'll rarely drive) and what isn't (e.g., longing to fulfill a dream). Review your friend's past to understand the behaviors. *What did he always want to do? What are his regrets? His dreams?* We move in a world created by our history and often pretend the past and present aren't connected. One of my most important unfulfilled dreams is being competent enough to play with a musical group. I bought three expensive Andean flutes in Peru and made arrangements to return the following year for an intensive week of lessons on how to play indigenous Andean wind instruments within a group of accomplished musicians. Some friends couldn't understand why a seventy-year-old would travel almost five thousand miles to engage in an activity more appropriate for someone half my age. Fortunately, my wife understands that this will be my last opportunity to fulfill a dream. My decision becomes understandable by knowing my history, including my losses.

Suggestions

14. Don't ignore the big picture when you try to understand your loved one's behaviors.
15. Assume that a behavior appears strange because you don't understand its meaning.
16. Don't use the context of a healthy person to understand the decisions of a person living with cancer.
17. Search for how the hidden meaning of behaviors is related to issues of closure.
18. Don't judge behaviors within a vacuum. Always assume they connect to the past.

ACCEPT CHANGES IN IDENTITY

Someone with a new diagnosis is still wrestling with a changing identity. This is a difficult time for your loved one regardless of her age.[10] How he views himself—his identity—is based on what he does; the roles he plays and the activities he enjoys; and his affiliations, values, abilities, and relationships. The person with cancer sees who he is now and compares the image to who he used to be and who he may become. A man in his seventies adored his young grandchildren. The highlight of every week was visiting with them, playing catch with his granddaughter and competing at video games with his grandson. The pain from throwing a ball or even moving a joystick became excruciating as the cancer spread. He lost his mobility and could only read, converse, and watch television with his grandchildren. He viewed himself as an old man waiting to die instead of being the playful grandfather his grandchildren adored. He knew he had changed, although his wife insisted he hadn't. "Funny Gramps," as his grandchildren called him, became "Gramps." He thought of himself as a different person because his interactions with his grandchildren had changed. His wife tried to reassure him that the grandchildren's love remained as strong as before the cancer. Instead of her assurances being helpful, he believed she wasn't giving legitimacy to how cancer was affecting his life.

To understand how many of us think of our "new" persona, imagine that someone drops you into a strange country with a language you don't understand and unfamiliar customs. I experienced a similar situation when I was in Prague in the Czech Republic and decided to drive to Weimer, Germany, a four-hour trip. I didn't speak Czech, and my German was as inadequate then as it was when I studied it in high school. In many ways, the person receiving a cancer diagnosis is on a similar journey. What she thought a life-threatening disease would be like wasn't close to what she actually experienced. Until you have cancer, everything is theoretical. Once a loved one learns of the diagnosis, what was theory becomes reality.

The person you knew for years doesn't appear to have changed after the diagnosis although the cancer may have taken away something significant in her life. An offhand but supportive comment you made about her hair loss (e.g., "You look good to me without hair") can be interpreted negatively rather than as a compliment. Cancer and its treatment take away treasured parts of our lives. Change one significant element and our identity changes. Losses are by-products of chronic and terminal illnesses.[11] It can be the daily jog for someone who ran for forty years, the loss of hearing for someone who played the cello her entire life, or the gradual memory loss of a writer who spent his days in front of a computer crafting short stories. A younger person who thought he had decades left may believe only a few years remain, despite his physician's assurance his cancer is curable. The older person who thought he was prepared to die after a fruitful life realizes his "thinking" about death is not the same as facing a limited future. I spent an afternoon talking with a dear colleague who was dying from pancreatic cancer. She had a full life, with wonderful adult children she adored and who adored her. For twenty years as a psychologist, she had influenced the lives of people she counseled, but her meaningful life hadn't prepared her for death. Despite knowing she had made a difference in many people's lives, she wondered whether her life had been purposeful enough. Don't expect consistency in how your friend approaches her illness. Assume that whatever stability was present in her life is undermined by the illness and that until she adjusts to her new condition, your life with her may be unsettling.

Think of cancer as a subtractive process, a malevolent entity taking away lifelong defining roles (e.g., sportsman, musician, activist). With progressive cancers, losses either accumulate within one realm of functioning (e.g., gradual reduction of strength) or become pervasive, touching multiple aspects of our life (e.g., sexual activity, strength, mental acuity). A mistake many people make is assuming that identities stabilize as the cancer and its treatment plateau. The reasoning is that once people adjust to the effects of treatment or the cancer's growth, changes will be minimal. Even if the cancer becomes stabilized and the treatment effects are predictable and short term, the assault on a person's body and psyche may continue. For example, although my cancer has been stable for the past thirteen years, I'm reminded daily of the losses caused by my treatments. The only thing certain about cancer and its treatment is its unpredictability.[12]

Suggestions

19. Changes in identity affect perceptions and behaviors.
20. Reassure your loved one of your continued support without minimizing the effects of cancer.
21. Changes in identity may not be stable. Identities change as losses accumulate.
22. Help your loved one adjust to her new identity rather than maintaining she's the same person she was before the diagnosis.
23. Think of cancer as a subtractive process.

5

CONVERSATIONS

" A whole chapter on conversations?" a reviewer of this chapter said. "Isn't this a book on supporting people living with cancer?" My answer was "Yes, but the unskillful use of words results in conflicts between a person living with cancer and loved ones." Most people believe they are skilled speakers, astute listeners, or both. You may think that comments to your loved one are always unambiguous and honest. She may have a different opinion. After years of research on how people communicate and listen, I concluded that we rarely view the world objectively.[1] What we see, hear, and communicate is often determined by our needs, beliefs, and history.

If someone asked "What is a conversation?" you may think about back-and-forth verbal interactions. One person says something, followed by a response from another person, and then the cycle is repeated until the conversation ends. Conversations are more complicated than back-and-forth verbal interactions. For example, you share something of great importance with your friend regarding an embarrassing moment. You stop and wait for her reaction. She proceeds to tell you what happened to her last week at work rather than asking how you felt. You wonder whether she's interested in what you experienced. We think of conversations as communications seamlessly ebbing and flowing, but an analysis of what's occurring within conversations reveals intricacies that shape attitudes and behaviors in strange ways.

WHY AND HOW TO ANALYZE CONVERSATIONS

Some people may view attempts to analyze conversations with loved ones and friends as artificial. You are asked to take something natural and look at it clinically. Further, you may believe the conscious manipulation of speech and language will destroy the ease and dynamics of your conversations. Arguments against using a conversational analysis with friends and loved ones ignore one basic purpose of conversations with loved ones who are coping with cancer: to provide compassionate support. In each of the following sections, one "hidden" aspect of conversations is explained. Think of them as eight "healthy" strategies for enhancing verbal interactions:

- Listen more and talk less
- Assure conversational flow
- Clearly express ideas
- Prevent message interference
- Reduce or eliminate hostility
- Make meanings clear
- Reduce anxiety levels
- Prevent a discrepancy between words and actions
- Look for hidden meanings

The sophistication of your analysis can range from a casual observer to what you'd expect from a university researcher.

Suggestions

1. A conversational analysis will enable you to understand how the style of your interaction affects your loved one.
2. Don't be concerned about the sophistication of your analysis. Simple is better than sophisticated and some is better than none.
3. Your analysis of the conversation can be short since there is consistency in how we communicate. A ten-minute sample is sufficient.

LISTEN MORE AND TALK LESS

Many people believe they can show support through words. Often the greatest support comes from silently witnessing what a person with cancer is experiencing. Ask yourself before you speak during those uncomfortable silent periods whether what you are about to say is necessary. Can your concerns be conveyed by your presence or touch or by holding a loved one's hand? At a workshop, Sogyal Rinpoche said lectures are for entertainment and silence for deep learning.[2] Ignoring the importance of silence was evident when a patient with prostate cancer visited his cousin. They never were close, but their relationship was continuous for many years. Each had been available for the other during various crises in their lives, so Jim hoped she could serve as a sounding board for his feelings. "Jim, you look great today," she said. Jim knew he wasn't looking better. He lost 20 percent of his body weight as the disease progressed and the cancer affected his digestive system. While he was composing his thoughts about the possibility of dying, the cousin said, "The weather is so mild today. Why don't we go out to the front porch and sit?" After waiting less than fifteen seconds for Jim to respond, she said, "Would you like to see some pictures of our trip to Europe?" She wasn't insensitive, but as with many people, silence for her was something uncomfortable and meant to be filled.[3] Think about how this interaction would have been different if she had remained quiet until Jim was ready to speak. Sometimes only a calm presence and compassionate listening are necessary.[4]

Silence becomes the breathing space in which people living with cancer can begin difficult conversations. A few years ago, a massive gas explosion devastated a neighborhood in San Bruno, a small town south of San Francisco.[5] My wife was asked to register evacuees at one of the Red Cross shelters. I accompanied her and, along with other volunteers, registered those who had survived the explosion and fire. Most people who came into the shelter appeared to be in shock and needed to talk. Many had run to safety as they watched homes on their block ignite. Others saw homes explode with occupants still inside. Interviewers who held to the Red Cross script got only the information the Red Cross sought. Those of us who listened and allowed periods of silence to be filled by what the survivors wanted to say heard descriptions of shocking events and expressions of terrifying emotions. For many, it was the first time they had spoken about their experiences. Even though we allowed them to talk as much as they wanted, by asking only a few questions, we got the information requested by the Red Cross. Sometimes the most emotionally relevant information will come during those periods when you may be struggling with what you can say to fill the silence.

Your loved one may be grappling with choices that have grave consequences. You hope she will find it easy to share her fears with you, but often a lifetime spent not showing vulnerabilities makes it difficult to be open. For two months, I spent every Friday with Bill, a man who was dying of hepatitis. We would drive to Lands End, a scenic place in San Francisco, and peer at the Golden Gate Bridge to our right and the Pacific Ocean to our left. It was a setting conducive to silence. Bill talked about his life as he smoked his medical marijuana. I wanted to ask for specifics but didn't want to interrupt him. We remained sitting on the bench until it was almost dark. During the three hours, I said little. When he had finished an idea, I gave him time to compose another. It was obvious he had a need to tell his story and share his fears about dying without my interrupting him or being judgmental.

Suggestions

4. Sometimes compassionate listening is more supportive than filling the silence with words.
5. Allow silence to be the breathing space in which your loved one prepares to share painful feelings or topics.
6. Don't interrupt and do be nonjudgmental.

ASSURE CONVERSATIONAL FLOW

We often don't listen to what is said to us, formulating responses before the person finishes expressing her thoughts. Our responses may not relate to what preceded them and, in some instances, distance us from the individual who is speaking. As a speech-language pathologist, I often analyzed conversations between parents and children—especially if parents suspected their child had a language problem.[6] While most parents were astute in realizing there was a problem, they didn't realize their style of interaction was contributing to it. One very common issue was their responses often had little to do with what their child was saying. Identical problems exist with adult conversations.

I found the same conversational approach useful when I began counseling people living with cancer and their caregivers.[7] A client with lung cancer told me about an interaction he had with his wife following a chemotherapy treatment. They were married for thirty years, and although he loved her, she had the annoying habit of not listening, preferring to change topics when she felt her needs or ideas were more important than her husband's needs. She was upset by a high bill from the utility company and ranted about the error until he said, "Dear, I have a problem breathing. Can we talk about this later?" She continued talking about the bill as if he had never said anything. Her anger with the utility company was so great that she couldn't hear the fear in her husband's voice. He believed she was placing an error of $30 over acknowledging his fear. It wasn't that she didn't care; rather, she was unaware of the impression she gave by not listening to what he said. She didn't see a connection between what she was saying and her husband's subsequent annoyance.

The idea of the unintended consequences of "connectedness" is illustrated by the belief that the flapping of a butterfly's wings in Africa can start a hurricane in the Atlantic Ocean. Whether this meteorological phenomena is true, conversations have similar unintended consequences.[8] I say something and you respond. I say something else and you respond, and so on and so forth. The joking comment you made last week about your husband's problems driving may become the background three weeks later for an unrelated conversation about his cancer. You thought your comment about his driving skills was a casual comment of little importance. Your husband interpreted it as displeasure that his cancer was inconveniencing you. Start with the assumption that connected statements give better results and greater bonding than successive monologues. You don't need to record, transcribe, and analyze your entire conversation. Listen to what your wife is saying. Make sure your response is directly related to her comment. Throughout your conversation, repeat the pattern. After the conversation ends, ask yourself how this conversation differed from others.

The direction conversations take is rarely set.[9] When I was still counseling, I was always aware of the sequence of statements in conversations with clients. I would anticipate what they would say and how I would respond, and then how they would respond to my response. After analyzing the interactions of hundreds of clients over a thirty-year period, I began to understand what moved conversations forward and what impeded them.[10] One of the most significant variables was whether the interaction consisted of successive monologues or a well-connected dialogue.[11] When one person dominates the conversation, the person doing the listening believes her concerns are deemed unimportant by the speaker.

There are consequences whether you are the person monopolizing the conversation or the person waiting his turn to speak. The speaker is announcing that "What I'm saying is so important, wait until I'm done talking before you speak." The listener, who feels she must fight to get in her comments, may view the person monopolizing the conversation as uncaring. An inequitable speaking-listening pattern affects relationships. Conversely, conversations where there is a balance between who speaks and who listens are bonding.[12] An important consequence of these types of conversations is that they indicate a solidarity in dealing with an issue. When your wife shares important information, her hope is that you are attentive to what she is saying, and that you'll place as much importance on it as she does. An indication you are giving it equal importance is often based on your first few responses. For example, if you and your wife are trying to determine how your lives will change because of the cancer, an interaction where each person listens to the other and comments on what was said rather than going off on another topic will be more positive than one with disjointed comments. Compare the two examples below.

Example 1:

> *Wife:* I think we need to change our plans for the Florida trip. I don't feel I'll be well enough to travel by then.
>
> *Husband:* I can understand your reluctance. What problems do you anticipate?
>
> *Wife:* I will have just stopped chemotherapy, and I don't think I'll be comfortable sitting on an airplane for six hours.
>
> *Husband:* I understand. Would you like to postpone it?

In the second example, the wife's statements remain the same, but the husband's change.

Example 2:

> *Wife:* I think we need to change our plans for the Florida trip. I don't feel I'll be well enough to travel by then.
>
> *Husband:* I already spent the money for the nonrefundable reservations.
>
> *Wife:* I will have just stopped chemotherapy, and I don't think I'll be comfortable sitting on an airplane for six hours.
>
> *Husband:* You chose chemotherapy rather than radiation and also when it would begin.

In example 1, the wife told her husband about her concerns, and in response he invited her to provide more details. He's saying her concerns are important and he wants her to lead the conversation. In example 2, the wife's concerns are subverted to the husband's financial issues. The husband's response implies that his wife's fears about her physical ability are secondary to his money concerns. Finances may be crucial for this couple, but there are better ways of introducing their importance without ignoring his wife's fear.

Another type of conversational flow problem occurs when someone is forced to answer questions rather than initiating topics. The first category of questions is "closed ended." These are questions requiring yes–no responses or specific answers to direct questions (e.g., "When is your next doctor's appointment?"). Think about the inquisitor role of old-time elementary school teachers, lawyers in a trial, police officers, and others who structure conversations based on question-and-answer interactions. The person on the receiving end is in the "hot seat." Question-and-answer interactions are appropriate for a police officer's investigation, but they can create defensive reactions if a loved one believes you are questioning the veracity of her comment. There are times when direct questions are necessary, but they shouldn't be the foundation on which you converse.

The second type of question is called "open ended" and often constitutes the bulk of a therapist's utterances in psychotherapy sessions. An example would be "Tell me how you felt when the doctor informed you of your cancer diagnosis." It provides the latitude for the individual who is answering to identify something important. Open-ended questions often produce significant insights for the person who poses them and the person answering them. Open-ended questions are better than closed-ended questions, but they shouldn't dominate your conversation. There is nothing wrong with asking questions, but to strengthen a relationship, fill your conversation with responses containing elaborations, relevant comments, and reiterations.[13]

Suggestions

7. Connect your comments directly to those of your loved one.
8. Be prepared to follow the conversation's trend.
9. Identify the type of statements moving a conversation forward and ones impeding it.
10. Use dialogues rather than successive monologues to develop bonding.
11. Allow your loved one to speak as much or more than you do.
12. Engage more in conversations and less in question-and-answer interactions.
13. If you are using a question format, try to keep the questions open ended rather than closed.

CLEARLY EXPRESS IDEAS

Content is considered the "meat" of conversations. Its presentation is analogous to a food's preparation. An expensive cut of Kobe beef becomes a piece of leather if it is not cooked properly. Likewise, the manner of presentation can destroy the intent of a message. There are many ways of analyzing how we express ideas. The most important involve intonation, word and sentence choice, and phrasing.

Intonation. Many years ago, when my daughter was a teenager, we were discussing a choice she had made that I thought was unwise. I tried to be supportive in my words despite disagreeing with her decision. I thought I was successful in hiding my concerns until she said, "It's not *what* you say, Daddy; it's *how* you say it." Given a choice between believing my words or my contradictory tone, there was no hesitation in choosing—the tone of my communications gave more information about my feelings than my words. Intonation refers to the qualities of intensity, pitch, register, tempo, duration, and tension.[14] Fact-checking uses intonation. *Are the words and intonation in sync, or, as with my lack of support for my daughter's choice, does my intonation pattern make my words less than truthful?*

Infants rely on intonation before they understand the meaning of words.[15] As adults, we rely on this early developed skill to check for the truth of a speaker's words.[16] Discrepancies between the meaning of words and their presentation are resolved by our mind favoring intonation patterns.[17] There will be times when you may be choosing your words to hide what you're feeling. You believe you can convey one idea while believing another, but your failures at hiding feelings will most likely exceed your successes. Researchers in the 1970s found that when there was a discrepancy between the message conveyed in words and the tone, listeners relied less on words and more on tone.[18] For example, using the phrase "I support your treatment decision," but conveying it through a neutral or negative intonation pattern, sends a qualified message to your loved one: *Don't believe his words—listen to how he says them.* The inability to monitor intonation extends to other nonverbal behaviors such as some facial expressions, arm and leg movements, and posture. Messages coming from nonverbal modalities have more credence than verbal messages.[19] So don't be shocked if your loved one interprets your support as being less than positive when your nonverbal behaviors qualify or negate your verbal message. Your loved one is more likely to rely on tone rather than words to evaluate your support when the two are disparate.[20]

You shouldn't "adjust" your tone to make it compatible with your words since monitoring tone for more than a few minutes is difficult.[21] If you know tone will "give you away," it might be better to forget trying to make the message conveyed by different modalities consistent and instead be honest. For example, you want to be supportive of a treatment option you disagree with so you try to modify your intonation, attempting to make it consistent with your words. Honesty would be a better approach to voice your concerns. For example, a father informs his son of a new treatment he believes will halt the cancer's progress. The son is familiar with the treatment and knows it is fraudulent. The father's medical team has exhausted all treatment protocols and informed him it might be time to get his affairs in order. The father's enthusiasm for a disproven approach may be a desperate attempt to avoid end-of-life issues. The son's intonation pattern when saying "I support your decision, Dad" will be interpreted as disapproval. A better approach would be for the son to support his father's choice while being honest about his feelings: "I support your choice, Dad, but I need to share with you how I feel about it." Select words offering support while still acknowledging your concerns instead of trying to make your intonation consistent with your words.

Choosing words and sentence structure. Your selection of words may result in unintended consequences. For example, when you need to shop, you say to your loved one "I'm going to the store." When you're exhausted, you say "I'm going to sleep for an hour." In both cases, you're expressing your legitimate needs. But what if your loved one expresses fear of being left alone even for a short period? How would your message be interpreted if you rephrased these sentences in the following way: *I need to go to the store. Will you be all right here alone for thirty minutes?* or *I'm exhausted, and I need to sleep for an hour. Is there anything I can do for you before I lie down?* Both examples convey information, but the revisions show sensitivity to your loved one's needs. Years ago, I served a woman with abdominal cancer in an extended care facility. I met her daughter during one of my visits. Between visits her mother had a stroke, making expressive communication difficult.[22] I needed to explain some communication strategies to the daughter. I said to the mother before we began the conversation, "I need to explain to your daughter some ways of communicating with you. I know you can hear us and understand everything we will be saying, even though you may have problems using words. Will it be all right if we speak about your condition even if you're not in the conversation?" My explanation may seem like a laborious unnecessary step, but it wasn't. I could have said, "I need to talk about your language problem to your daughter now" or even said nothing about excluding her and began the conversation with the daughter. Sometimes, the addition of a few words acknowledging your loved one's needs can do much to convey your compassion, even when you believe the message is informational.

Your message may be easier to focus on if you use less complex words and simpler grammar.[23] It has nothing to do with neurology unless the brain has been affected by the cancer. Given a limited amount of attentive ability, the more your loved one can focus on the content of a message, the more likely she'll receive it accurately. Complex sentence structures and ten-dollar words make attending to a message more difficult. I had a patient who had grown up in Oklahoma during the Depression. His family had lived on a subsistence farm and since times were bad none of the children had gone to school. They had worked the fields from early morning until the sun set. My patient had taught himself to read during nonwork hours. The ideas he expressed were worthy of being said by a social philosopher: observations about life, theories of governance, and how he was trying to get past the racial bigotry inculcated in him by a rural Oklahoma society of the 1930s. All were expressed using simple words and linguistic structures typical of someone in grade school.

"You know," he said, "I'm only comfortable talking to you and the nurse."

"Why?"

"Both of you use words I understand. Some of the other people who come to the house use words I never heard."

"Do you ask them what they mean?"

"No, never. If I did, they would know I never had any schooling. And then what would they think about me?"

He listened to important information he didn't understand and remained silent so not to appear "stupid." His wife, who was disabled by a stroke, couldn't help, since she had limited comprehensive ability. He misunderstood medicine dosages, didn't access financial assistance for paying utilities, and lacked an understanding of how hospice worked. These problems didn't result from any cognitive deficit but rather from the embarrassment of not knowing the meaning of some words. Choosing a simpler way to communicate doesn't mean your loved one has lost the ability to understand complexities. Rather, global changes are making it harder to process information. Think about a computer whose memory is maxed out because of additional programs you loaded. Searches still work and software programs can still be accessed. But everything slows down. Your loved one can focus on your intended message if you keep words simple and choose uncomplicated linguistic structures.

Phrasing. How annoyed do you become at a presentation when the speaker links an endless string of ideas as if they are seamless? Seven ideas pass while you struggle to comprehend the first idea. The processing of verbal information is complex.[24] If speakers understand this, sales people trying to convince you to buy a product will break up their presentation into bite-size ideas, punctuated with breaks. For example, if you are attempting to convince your loved one it would be beneficial to try a new intervention procedure, you would present only one idea or a few ideas for him to process before inserting a break into your message since more time is needed to process incoming information under stressful conditions.[25] When a speaker chunks ideas together, the effect of the first is reduced if the listener is trying to comprehend the second, and vice versa.[26] It's a good practice to pause between ideas. The more ideas presented without an opportunity to process them, the more likely your loved one may misinterpret or ignore some of them. For example, here are two different ways of presenting the same idea. Read each example out loud and choose the style you prefer.

Example 1:

> The doctor suggested that you try this new medication for four days a week so your liver has a chance to heal following the radiation treatment that is affecting its ability to produce proteins necessary for blood clotting.

Example 2:

> The doctor suggested a new medication.
> (pause)
> He would like you to try it for four days a week.
> (pause)
> If it works, it will give your liver a chance to produce proteins necessary for blood clotting.

Our minds turn themselves off when the information we are trying to comprehend exceeds our processing capabilities.[27] When we experience an overload, instead of listening, we dream, focus on a person sitting in front of us, or maybe even decide what we will cook for dinner. Anything to avoid overloading our exhausted minds with strings of ideas having no breaks. Don't restrict your conversations to "one idea, one phrase." You can hear the effect of this in the speech of politicians such as Republican presidential candidate Ted Cruz, whose consistent use of "one idea, one phrase" introduces an artificiality into his speech. Save this valuable technique for critical ideas, not casual conversations.

Go slowly. Drugs, pain, medication, and dealing with a new or uncertain status can increase processing time.[28] One of the simplest techniques you can use to enhance comprehension is to slow your speech. Many people believe "slow speech" is a useful tactic only with people whose cognitive abilities are impaired (e.g., Alzheimer's and other forms of dementia). I don't view myself as cognitively impaired, yet fast speech taxes my comprehension ability. For example, I dread calling a customer service department. I know the likelihood is high that the agent will be located offshore and that he or she will speak with a pronounced accent and use a speaking rate of more than two hundred words per minute. Why is this a problem? Thirty percent of people over sixty-five have a hearing loss affecting comprehension, as I do.[29] The problem is greater over the telephone than it is when speaking in person. I need more processing time at seventy than I did at forty, as do most older people.[30] I know I will miss much of what is said as the representative's speaking rate increases. One would think that as a speech-language pathologist, I could understand accented speech better than a non-speech-language pathologist, but I can't. With impaired hearing I often ask the representatives to repeat or slow down. No matter how hard they try to slow their rate, I know within a few minutes it will approach the one neurologically set.[31]

Loved ones with normal hearing may have similar problems. With a hearing impairment and an aging brain, I have difficulty attending to some messages. Your loved one's difficulty in listening may come from physical pain or psychological stress. I try to keep my speech around one hundred words per minute when I'm counseling clients. The rate reduction may not be necessary for some clients, but I never know the range of issues with which they are dealing or whether there is a hearing problem or an age-related processing problem. The effects on comprehension can be dramatic if you can drop from two hundred words a minute to under one hundred. If this 50 percent rate reduction is too difficult to maintain or sounds strange to your loved one, drop your rate in smaller increments, say going from 200 words a minute to 175, then to 150, and finally to under 100.

Actions are better than words. Never miss the opportunity to express your compassion through the use of words, but when possible express your compassion through actions. The actions don't need to involve huge gestures. They can be small, similar to the one I witnessed in a hospice with a man in his nineties. He had been a patient for two months and during the entire time confined to his bed. His world was limited to his frontal and peripheral vision. When a volunteer noticed the patient was fascinated with the few birds landing in the branches outside his window, he purchased an inexpensive bird feeder and installed it while the patient slept. Upon wakening the patient found several birds on the feeder. The daily visits of the birds expanded the patient's world and was the highlight of his last months of life. The volunteer's placement of the bird feeder said more to the patient about the love the volunteer had for him than any words he ever could have expressed. Expressions of your compassion are stronger through little things having immediate consequences rather than words or the occasional grand gesture. "Show, don't tell" is an idea taught to aspiring writers of fiction. Transform the concept into "Do, don't just say."

Suggestions

14. Intonation will be used to determine your feelings if your words and intonation don't match.
15. Discuss your concerns instead of hiding your feelings by monitoring your intonation, since hiding the discrepancy will most likely be unsuccessful.
16. Use simple grammatical structures and words even if your loved one's cognitive ability is normal.
17. Minimize the number of ideas within each phrase for important issues.
18. Compensate for the effects of drugs, medications, and emotional problems by slowing speech, but not to where it sounds abnormal.
19. Your choice of words should account for your loved one's physical and emotional needs.

PREVENT MESSAGE INTERFERENCE

What is noise? The answer depends on a person's history and current living conditions.[32] To someone who lives in rural areas, the hum of a car's tires on a smooth road might be considered noise. To an urban dweller living in the country, crickets produce an unbearable racket. Noise, for the communications specialist, is anything interfering with receiving or delivering a message.[33] Noise often has little to do with loudness; rather, it's anything disruptive to your loved one's ability to attend or think. For someone coping with the effects of chemotherapy, it could be construction noises echoing on the street, the laughter of children from an apartment next door, the spewing of commercials from a television in the next room, or even the babble of people trying to talk simultaneously in her presence. A man recovering from lung surgery complained that his grandchildren's play activity was disruptive. Even after the children had heeded their father's instructions to "tone it down because Grandpa isn't feeling well," the grandfather felt no relief. The son believed that his father's criticism of his grandchildren was unwarranted since the children went from yelling to talking quietly. What the son didn't realize was that his father's annoyance had little to do with the volume of his grandchildren's speech. Rather, it was the presence of anything affecting his ability to focus on his cancer.

Noise is also thought to be calming by some family and professional caregivers. I served a woman in a nursing home with overworked staff. With not enough caregivers for the number of patients, the staff and administrators believed continuous television shows would provide a distraction to reduce residents' requests. When I visited, the volume of the television at the foot of my patient's bed was so loud that I had to take out my hearing aids. Stepping out into the hallway, I heard other televisions blaring, many tuned to different stations. The cacophony of sounds reminded me of an airport with simultaneous announcements and distorting echoes. The staff members were pleased with the results. They told me that since the introduction of the policy the number of patient requests had decreased by 30 percent. The strategy was effective for reducing patient demands, but it was disruptive to patients trying to deal with the effects of their illnesses.

Noise can be neutral regarding intention (it's just there), used as a way of minimizing the effect or discomfort of a person's distress (block out depressing thoughts), or as was the case at the nursing home, inappropriate. Don't assume that your loved one wants to be distracted. Always ask whether it's all right before turning on a television, radio, or a CD player. *Always* turn off all media when you begin an important conversation. For loved ones coping with cancer and its treatment effects, noise, regardless of its source, interferes with the sorting out of thoughts. Trying to think about something important while *The Price Is Right* is playing on the TV or a Mozart opera plays in the background is difficult if not impossible. For some people the presence of noise is a minor nuisance. Research shows that we adapt to some noises in a short amount of time by relying on a neurological filter to suppress disruptive sounds.[34] These filters are less effective when a person is dealing with a substantial problem. To understand the effects of noise, turn on a television and try having a substantive conversation with your loved one. Increase the volume if the sound doesn't pose a problem, and continue your conversation. At some point, you will reach a volume level where a meaningful conversation becomes impossible. A different kind of problem occurs when your loved one insists that a distraction remain during an important communication. Assume one of two things: The topic is frightening, and noise is one way of reducing its effect, as was the case with a woman who knew she needed chemotherapy but watched daytime soap operas to avoid thinking about it. The second is when the need for distraction involves broad issues, as was the case with a client who wanted to reduce the effect of conversations related to changes in his identity. He had been a salesperson his entire life, relying on his ability to be glib for selling products. His identity changed with the losses he experienced related to thyroid cancer. He insisted on watching TV whenever his wife wanted to discuss his cancer. "Not now, dear; let me just finish this episode," was a frequently used statement to avoid discussing his feelings. If you think your loved one is using noise as a distraction, begin a conversation about her fears rather than arguing about noise.

Suggestions

20. Minimize noise.
21. Don't use noise for distraction.
22. Always turn off all media during important conversations.
23. Your loved one's insistence that a noise source remains can be an indication she fears dealing with the topic or wants to mute her feelings.

THE IMPORTANCE OF TIMING

Few people look forward to discussing anything frightening. The possibility of dying from cancer or deciding how to cope with it ranks close to the top. What's difficult to determine is when the time is right to begin discussions involving disability, a changing lifestyle, a new identity, difficult treatment options, and end-of-life issues. For one of my clients, the route was tortuous. Jim's doctor told him and his wife that his bladder cancer was treatable but the prognosis uncertain. He accepted the news in the doctor's office as if he had just learned he had a minor skin condition, but when he and his wife returned home, he was despondent. "I know this is frightening for you," his wife said. "I'm scared too. I want you to know when you're ready to talk, I'm here." She sat next to him and instead of forcing him to begin the conversation, held his hand and compassionately witnessed his emotional pain. She understood that a conversation wouldn't be useful while he was in emotional shock. The next day, he talked about a planned two-year house remodeling project as if the prognosis had never occurred. She didn't argue with him about the wisdom of proceeding with the remodel. It was apparent to her that he wasn't ready to talk about the possibility of dying, and until he was, she would wait. Three weeks later he said, "Let's talk about the prognosis. I didn't believe the physician when he told me about my odds of surviving. Now, my body is telling me it's time to deal with it."

If his wife had tried to have the conversation when her husband was in emotional shock, it could have resulted in a defensive reaction. Forcing a loved one or friend to "face reality," whether it involves the acceptance of a chronic illness or her impending death, rarely is fruitful; rather it creates additional anxiety.[35] Getting the timing right for a critical discussion is often the key for accepting the consequences of cancer.

Suggestion

24. Don't force difficult discussions. Wait until your loved one is ready.

LOOK FOR HIDDEN MEANINGS

Many years ago, I saw a black and white photograph taken by Richard Avedon in 1947 of a young Sicilian boy.[36] "Noto, Sicily" was the title of the photograph and the name of the Sicilian town where he took it. A teenage boy appears in the foreground, smiling and wearing a suit too short in the arms and too tight in the waist. In the background—softly out of focus—is a tree with a symmetrical oval canopy and a fence defining the boundary between sky and water. It is a bucolic scene, until you look at the boy. His ill-fitting suit has little to do with parents who can't afford to buy the correct size. Rather, the boy's body is racked with deformities: a humped back, emaciated legs, and a chest out of proportion to his body. What appears to be obvious isn't. Many of our behaviors, as was the boy's appearance, aren't what they seem.

To understand your loved one's communications, peer behind what you think is obvious. He may wish to spare you knowing of the physical pain he's experiencing or the emotional turmoil of living with cancer. Most utterances have functions. Three common ones are descriptive, directive, and imperative. An example of a descriptive statement is when a loved one says, "I'm exhausted. I'd like to sleep now." A directive statement would be "Please get me the blanket; I'm cold." An example of an imperative remark would be "It's wonderful to feel so good without the pain!" These functions are easy to understand. The problem arises when there is a hidden meaning to the utterance, as occurred with a father who spent his life trying to meet his wife's and daughter's needs. He always anticipated their problems, and as his cancer became more active, he assumed they would anticipate his needs. When they didn't, his interactions with them became negative. While the words were neutral, his intonation pattern was hostile. Eventually, his wife realized something was annoying him. If you suspect that your loved one is communicating a message with a hidden meaning, don't speculate. Ask him want he means.

Suggestion

25. Don't speculate on the hidden meaning. Explain to your loved one you need more clarification.

6

DISCOMFORT, PAIN,
AND SUFFERING

The terms "discomfort," "pain," and "suffering" refer to the same phenomena—an unwelcome physical experience or emotional feeling.
What differentiates the three from each other is the length of time your
loved one experiences each and its intensity. Medication can be a blessing
for pain and suffering one day and inconsequential the next. There is jubilation when the pain stops or becomes manageable, but the fear the reprieve
will end tempers joy. On bad days, your loved one may fear the pain will
never relent and become a feature dominating her life. We think of pain
as bounded by a beginning and an end point, but the emotional aspects
of pain are porous, affecting thinking not only during the experience but
before and after the pain stops. You can use a distraction to reduce the intensity of the pain, but you may be limited to compassionately witnessing
it. Your loved one can learn from discomfort, pain, or suffering, but avoid
suggesting anything positive in the experience when it is occurring.

MEDICATION

There is more artistry than science in finding the appropriate amount of
pain medication.[1] Your loved one can be overmedicated to where he isn't
aware of his surroundings, or at the other end of the continuum, an inadequate dose may have minimal effect on the pain. The difficulty for medical
personnel is finding the midpoint, where the medicine controls the pain
and the person still maintains awareness.[2] Physicians take two approaches:
start with a minimal dosage and work their way up until the pain becomes
acceptable or start with the maximum dosage and work their way down
until awareness is acceptable while minimizing the pain.[3] Don't be surprised

that if given an option your loved one chooses to take the maximum allowable dosage. She may not wish to wait until a pain threshold has been crossed, or she may prefer oblivion to waiting for the physician to find the appropriate dosage. We often equate the need for painkillers with intense pain, but as I discovered with one client, it's often used for other reasons. A physician prescribed marijuana for a patient to reduce nausea and pain associated with liver cancer. Once when I was with him and he was smoking, I asked him whether I could do anything to help him with the pain. "What pain?" he said. I explained that since he was using marijuana, I assumed he was in pain. "Pain can take many forms," he said. He went on to explain that even when the pain was minimal and he experienced only discomfort, marijuana allowed him to escape the constant awareness that he was dying. "Sometimes I just need to be stoned."

The possibility of addiction to opiates is minimal if they are used to manage pain from cancer under the supervision of a palliative care specialist.[4] Hospitals use a 0–10 pain management continuum for patients to self-report their pain.[5] Zero is none and ten is unbearable. Pain is subjective. An identical minor bruise for two people can be described as "not a problem" for one person and "excruciating" for another because the way in which the body interprets an assault goes beyond physical problems.[6] The correct pain number is the number your loved one gives you. Think of the self-assessment as having two critical features. The first is that the pain number acts as a reference point for requesting future medication. For example, a patient asks for medicine when she describes her pain reaching a 6 level. The reference number in future pain events then becomes 6 when you or a medical professional provides medication. The pain number also becomes the benchmark for determining the course pain takes.[7] For example, if your loved one reports a 2 at 2:00 p.m., a 3 at 2:25 p.m. and a 5 at 2:45 p.m., you can conclude that the pain is on the rise and medication is needed. Pain is easier to control when ascending rather than after having leveled off or before it becomes intolerable. A maxim used in palliative care is to attack early and adequately. More medication is required if you wait until the pain is unbearable, and it may take longer to manage.[8] An additional benefit of adequate pain control is its enhancing healing effect.[9]

Wait to give medication when the pain is descending and tolerable. Conversely, when ascending, provide an adequate level of medication to control or reduce it. No matter what you observe, always seek guidance from medical personnel who are experts in pain management.

In the late 1990s, there was an outcry that physicians were not prescribing enough opiates to control pain.[10] The medical community cited many reasons for the underuse, ranging from not understanding the effectiveness of opioids to outdated governmental regulations. Studies found that addiction to opioids was nonexistent if they were appropriately prescribed to relieve cancer pain.[11] The abuse of opiates increased as the number of prescriptions rose, especially hydrocodone and controlled-release (CR) oxycodone.[12] Much of the research on opiates found addiction to be a problem with chronic nonmalignant pain but not with cancer-related pain.[13]

For some people, such as a husband of a woman I counseled, fear of dependency because of an earlier alcoholism problem meant living with pain. Although a palliative care expert accounted for his past addiction when he made the dosage recommendations, my client would use only half of the prescribed opiate dosage when the pain became too intense.[14] His decision resulted in a minimal reduction of the pain.

Suggestions

1. Accept a loved one's decision to start with the maximum prescribed dosage.
2. Addiction rarely occurs in the management of cancer-related pain.
3. Use a hospital-based 0–10 pain management continuum and accept the number your loved one provides.
4. Track the increase or decrease of pain using the 0–10 continuum.

TREATING DISCOMFORT

Recently, the relationship between discomfort and opiate addiction has been getting attention.[15] Living with cancer is complicated. There may be times when your loved one tosses away the fear of addiction in preference for oblivion. Sometimes the psychological effects of discomfort can be as debilitating as pain. Unfortunately, physicians consider discomfort as something low level and either not requiring medication at all or requiring medication with only minimal analgesic properties. We have all experienced discomfort that we dismissed as temporary and annoying.

I had hoped the "don't be concerned" approach would apply to my oral surgery. The surgeon said I would experience more discomfort than pain. I knew the treatment of my cancer might complicate oral surgery since the bone structure available for implants was limited. In anticipation of the surgical outcome, the oral surgeon wrote a prescription for Vicodin. I explained that as a past hospice volunteer I was familiar with the palliative principles of pain control and that I would use the Vicodin only as the pain ascended. For the first week I limited my use of Vicodin to those times when I could tell the pain was increasing and had finally reached a 6 on the pain continuum. By the second week, the pain rarely reached a level I thought warranted medication. But by midafternoon, my jaw was exhausted from talking and eating. The discomfort of a 3 didn't warrant the use of opiates, but forgoing them made the remainder of the day miserable. By the third week, I began using Vicodin to provide a break from the constant discomfort I experienced from 3:00 p.m. until I went to sleep. I tossed out the palliative care warnings and took Vicodin to provide four to five hours of physical and emotional relief. I'm sure substance abuse experts would question my decision to use an opiate for "discomfort," since its use for discomfort is inappropriate and can lead to addiction. Your loved one may be tempted to use opiates or alcohol to stop an uncomfortable but not painful physical problem or emotional concern.

When she requests medication when she's not in pain, ask why she needs opiates. Your role in the management of pain and discomfort is not that of a narcotics agent but rather as someone who is willing to understand how physical or psychological discomfort can lead a loved one to believe medication is necessary. Discomfort can be short term (e.g., a few months), as when incisions are healing; have a longer duration, as it did with my oral surgery; or in some cases, last indefinitely. We often minimize discomfort when compared to pain or suffering. After all, the argument goes, isn't a little discomfort better than allowing a potentially deadly cancer to remain untreated? The "better than" scenario hides the effects of long-term discomfort. The discomfort from the oral surgery lasted for only four months. Even though the discomfort was a daily occurrence, I had a "discomfort-free" hiatus when I laid down and didn't eat or talk. But what if the discomfort is constant, as with a client whose surgery to remove a cancerous growth in his abdomen resulted in months of discomfort? The surgery saved his life, but the slightest movement for the next six months resulted in constant discomfort that led him to self-medicate with drugs and alcohol. "Pain is relative," he said to me. "There are times during the day when I want to experience life without discomfort. If that requires getting loaded from drugs or alcohol, so be it. I think I would go insane if I didn't have a break."

There are no easy answers for how to balance the need to stop discomfort with the possibility of creating an opiate addiction. Your loved one might find the inappropriate use of opiates to be an acceptable path if he believes he will be uncomfortable for a long time or forever. Discuss these types of decisions with palliative care experts. To understand his dilemma, imagine a pebble enters your boot during an all-day hike. While mildly annoying, you'll have to tolerate the discomfort for hours because the steep terrain doesn't have surfaces level enough to remove your boot. The peaceful hike you envisioned now becomes an ordeal. The analogy applies to your loved one, who knows the discomfort she is experiencing from the cancer or its treatment will last not hours but rather months or years. Does she tolerate the discomfort or opt for addictive drugs?

Suggestions

5. Mild long-term discomfort can have the same psychological effect as chronic pain.
6. Opiates are abused to reduce the psychological effects of discomfort.
7. Accept the legitimacy of discomfort as a debilitating condition requiring nondrug methods.

TREATING CHRONIC PAIN

What would you do if you learned, as one client did, that for the next six months you would be in pain? Not something mild like an occasional headache but something that overwhelms your thoughts, feelings, and behaviors. Some books maintain that with sufficient focus, the mind can conquer pain. I'm not sure whether any of the authors had sat with people in excruciating pain or experienced it themselves. I read a book written by a well-known awareness advocate, who wrote that a person could with practice separate herself from the pain she was experiencing. The problem with many of these books that espouse similar views on pain management is that they present a picture of what someone who is experiencing pain *should* be able to do rather than what they are actually capable of doing. I rarely saw evidence when I was a hospice volunteer that the mind could quell chronic pain for more than a short amount of time. You may find instances in your past where efforts to control pain with your mind were successful. But could you use the technique for six months? If you're like most people, instead of mind control you would rely on opiates.[16] For many people with chronic pain, predictability may be an elusive state of being. One day, the illness is controlled either by medication or an unknown factor, and the next day the pain comes on with the power of a sledgehammer. On good days, although there's jubilation, there's also the fear the reprieve will end. On bad days, there's the fear the pain will persist and never relent.

Suggestions

8. Don't expect long-term relief from mind control.
9. Chronic pain will affect everything your loved one experiences.
10. The occurrence of chronic pain is not predictable.

REDUCE SUFFERING

"Pain" is different from "suffering." Cassell made one of the first distinctions between the two. Suffering, he maintained, was distress going beyond physical pain, a state of being caused by a loss of integrity, intactness, cohesiveness, or the wholeness of the person.[17] A woman suffered from her husband's reactions to her cancer. Their relationship had been intimate, whether it involved sex or just the exchange of information sitting at dinner talking about the day's events. Everything changed when she had a mastectomy. Her husband said he couldn't deal with the "disfigurement" of her body. Their relationship deteriorated, and they went from sleeping in separate rooms with few conversations to a divorce. Her physical pain was manageable within a year after surgery, but she still suffered ten years later from her husband's rejection. I think physicians and even oncologists ignore the distinction between pain and suffering. I see "suffering" as a state of mind created when a person believes the dreadful emotion or pain he is experiencing will continue indefinitely. Suffering can be related either to physical pain or emotional trauma. A gentleman I served in hospice had prostate cancer with metastasis in his bones. His oncologist told him that while narcotics would help, they couldn't take away the pain. He would be in pain until he died. By not having a termination point, the pain became suffering. Unending "suffering" goes beyond physical pain. The emotional trauma caused by past unskillful acts may exceed the suffering linked to the cancer. One woman with cervical cancer disapproved of her son's choice of a wife, and as a result, she never met her grandchildren. The pain from the cancer was manageable, but she suffered from the effects of her thirty-year-old decision.

Suggestions

11. Differentiate pain from suffering.
12. Suffering can be emotional or physical.
13. You will want to stop the suffering but may be limited to compassionate witnessing.

THE BOUNDARIES OF PAIN ARE POROUS

We would like to think that pain has a beginning and an end point. For example, your loved one's pain starts around 9:00 a.m. when she starts moving, following a restful night, and ends by 1:00 p.m. when the medicine becomes active. Those of us who live with pain understand boundaries are porous. A patient said to me "I never know how long the pain will last, nor when it will begin again. No matter what I'm doing, I'm either waiting for it to go away or to start." When we see relief, we're thankful the event is over. But as another patient said, "Even when the pain isn't present, I fear its return." I had a client whose colorectal cancer was manageable. By "manageable," I mean the presence of pain was controllable: not enough pain to be debilitating but enough that he was aware of its presence. He had learned the signs of an approaching episode and took his medication. His wife assumed that being in control of the pain made life easier for her husband. Physically it did, but the thought of having to endure even a minimal amount of pain was psychologically debilitating. Although he was mobile, he limited his movements outside of the house since he never knew when the pain would return. His fear of the pain resulted in his eliminating activities that he had enjoyed his entire life, and since he couldn't predict when the pain would arrive, he shortened other activities.

How can pain be such a pervasive phenomenon even when absent? Sometimes the anticipation of pain is more debilitating than the pain itself.[18] Neurological studies show many of the same areas of the brain lighting up under pain are active when a person anticipates it.[19] I learned the role of anticipation after the hip replacement. I knew once my nonoperated leg was in bed, I would have to lift the operated one. I wasn't feeling any pain standing next to the bed, but I anticipated the agony I was about to experience. The reverse happened when I got out of bed. The pain lasted only a few seconds, but my anxiety continued as long as I anticipated it. I knew using the toilet would require at least four steps, each of which would result in pain: getting out of bed, sitting on the toilet, rising off the seat, and getting back into bed. I changed my eating habits to minimize bathroom trips. I doubt that the time in pain exceeded three minutes. I was amazed that only a few minutes of pain every day could have such an effect on my daily activities. Imagine your loved one making a decision to do something that she understands will cause immense pain but it's something required dozens of times a day. I knew that the intense pain would dissipate in a month and I'd look back at my recovery as a distant event. Your loved one's pain may remain indefinitely.

Suggestions

14. Treatment of pain goes beyond its beginning and end points.
15. Expect pain to affect your loved one's activities even when it's absent.
16. Discuss with your loved one what you can do to restructure her environment to reduce the pain.

THINKING DURING PAIN

Our first thoughts are to offer suggestions or solutions when a loved one experiences pain. When she rejects them, you may wonder why. Unless you have experienced intense pain, you may not understand how it can affect your ability to accept suggestions.[20] I learned about the power of pain when I awoke at midnight, believing my abdomen was about to explode. I didn't realize I was having a severe reaction to Vicodin for pain that was associated with a rotator cuff operation and unrelated to my cancer. A little Pepto-Bismol, I thought, and I'd be fine. But thirty minutes later I wasn't okay. I began having difficulty breathing and almost passed out as the intensity of the pain increased and spread. "Should we go to the emergency room?" my wife asked. I'm sure she expected me to say, "Let's wait 15 minutes," since I was always reluctant to seek medical attention. "No, call 911," I said in a whisper. After dressing and stumbling down the stairs, I lay on the couch waiting for the ambulance and thought I was dying. I had been present when patients died, and I often wondered how I would face death. Would there be any revelations or, as my atheistic friends predicted, "vast nothingness." Neither revelations nor darkness was present. Pain consumed me, and for the first time, I understood what many of my patients experienced. The pain obliterated the grand ideas I thought would be present as I approached death. I understand why some interrogators favor pain or its threat for obtaining information. I would have said anything while I was experiencing the pain to stop it—whether the information I provided was true or not. Your loved one may not have options for stopping her pain, or the options available may be inadequate. Don't try to have a rational conversation while she is experiencing intense pain.

Suggestion

17. Don't expect clarity of thought when your loved one is experiencing intense pain.

USE DISTRACTION TO MINIMIZE PAIN

A loved one will appreciate distractions if the cancer or its treatment causes pain. Don't expect to eliminate pain through distraction; rather, focus on reducing its impact by diverting attention with activities requiring minimal concentration.[21] Examples include listening to music, watching an intriguing movie not requiring much thought, or listening to someone tell a simple story, to mention a few. My most useful tool when I was in hospice was music. I was often asked to play my Native American flute and Shakuhachi for patients whose pain couldn't be controlled by medicine or who were in discomfort. I am at best a mediocre flutist, and I was concerned my playing would be more annoying than the pain patients were experiencing. One patient was semiconscious when I entered the room. I interpreted the tension on her face as the expression of pain. For a week, I had rehearsed a series of songs I hoped would give a patient some relief. As I started to play, I realized that staying with a set of memorized tunes would result in mistakes. There are few things as annoying as listening to a beautiful piece and having a discordant note ruin the mood the song was intended to create. Instead of adhering to my list of songs, I focused on playing improvised pieces. I could see her tension receding as I played, and after fifteen minutes she appeared peaceful. I saw similar effects when I played for other patients who were experiencing pain.

I knew the effect of the music had little to do with the quality of my musicianship. There was something about the music itself that helped reduce the pain. The literature is equivocal on the effectiveness of music to reduce pain. The problem according to researchers is that most studies are qualitative, with little objective data.[22] However, other studies suggest that music can lessen the sensation of pain, even if data are missing.[23] From my observations of how patients react to music, I believe the most significant variables are playing softly, using small transitions between notes, staying in major keys, and starting with low notes and ending with higher upbeat ones. I looked at the literature on pain and cognition to understand the effectiveness of what I was doing.[24] What I read corresponded to what I had seen with countless patients. Distraction requires patients to shift their focus from pain to unique sets of auditory or visual stimuli.

I asked one patient who found my playing helpful (not everyone did) why the music reduced her pain. She said, "It took me to a calm place where I still felt the pain, but I could tolerate it." The music should not require much thought, should pull the listener forward, and should be positive enough to affect the negativity of the pain. The same guidelines apply to other distracting methods. Simple positive stories with forward-moving themes are effective. Recorded music should follow the same principles of live music, and movies should require just enough cognition to follow the story line. I incorporated the principles of distraction for a patient with ALS whose stomach port became irritated and caused him pain, especially following a feeding. Since he was a great Abbott and Costello fan, we would cue up one of their routines. As soon as the pain began we would turn on the video, he would silently laugh as we watched "Who's on First?"

Think about the subjective experience of pain as a runaway car without brakes going down a hill. The occupants' fear builds as the car develops speed, consuming every thought they have. The same thing happens with pain. While people can still function at lower levels as the pain increases, everything else is blocked out. A mistake some people make is using distractions in place of pain medication. I saw the substitution work with only one person, who was a life-long meditator. At the onset of pain, she would begin meditating. Sometimes the technique was successful, but usually she would request medication during her meditation. Meditation, according to her, reduced the amount of pain medication she needed.

Suggestions

18. Distractions may minimize pain but not eliminate it.
19. Find activities that require minimal concentration.
20. Use the following principles if you play live or recorded music: play softly, keep the transitions between notes small, and look for songs starting with low notes and ending with higher ones.
21. Distracting activities should not require much thought, should pull your loved one forward, and should be positive enough to affect the negativity of the pain.

ACCEPT SUDDEN CHANGES IN PLANS

Nobody wants to do physical or social activities when he is anticipating or experiencing pain. A husband and wife were known to be the most social couple in their circle of friends. Dinners, parties, and various social events filled their calendar. When the husband developed lymphoma, he asked his wife to cancel many of their social commitments. His wife didn't object to canceling. She understood the toll the cancer was taking on her husband. What galled her was he often asked her to cancel only hours before the event. She didn't understand why he couldn't anticipate a problem when he accepted the date. She didn't factor in hope in her husband's decision. Despite knowing the possibility of attending an event was small, he hoped he could attend. The same dynamics existed with another client who defined his life by the activities he did with his grandchildren. Despite advancing problems with his cancer, every time his son and daughter-in-law asked him to visit, he said yes and canceled hours or minutes before the event. His hope that he could be with his grandchildren led him to accept the invitation, despite knowing the probability of his visit was minimal.

Acknowledge that you understand why a friend is canceling, and express a willingness to stay with her instead of going to a scheduled event. Your commitment will mitigate feelings of isolation. Also, plan activities that can be done even in the presence of pain. A client canceled outings with friends more because of the anticipation of pain than the actual pain. With each cancellation, her friends became more distant, eventually stopping efforts to include her in social events. A loved one is sending an explicit and implicit message when she cancels. The explicit message is easy to understand: *I'm not feeling well enough to do this.* The implicit message is more obscure: *I'm willing to risk isolation rather than do something painful.* You can mitigate feelings of isolation by staying with your loved one rather than attending the event despite her insistence that you leave her. You are saying your commitment to your loved one is greater than any enjoyment you would receive by leaving her alone. Your decision sends your loved one a powerful message.

Suggestions

22. Changes in plans and cancellations often are caused by more than one problem.
23. Expect hope at being able to attend an event to exceed her physical or emotional ability.
24. If your loved one cancels an event, offer to stay with her despite her insistence you go by yourself.
25. Schedule visits and possible events even if your loved one anticipates the presence of pain.
26. Acknowledge the legitimacy of your loved one's reasons for canceling.

DON'T ROMANTICIZE PAIN

Don't try to convince your loved one that she can learn anything from pain. Pain can be instructive, as I learned many times throughout my life, but people who have had the experience, including me, would prefer to remain ignorant. Twenty years ago I did a short retreat at the Shasta Abbey Buddhist Monastery. The year before I arrived, the Abbess, Reverend Master Jiyu-Kennett died of cancer.[25] An attending novice spoke of overhearing her each night before going to bed thanking the Buddha for giving her one more day to achieve enlightenment. The Abbess, according to him, was using the intense pain she experienced as a way of learning about life. For someone whose life revolved around spirituality, her ability and desire to learn from her pain was understandable. I think a friend who experiences pain would prefer a lucid conversation with you over a bottle of a thirty-year-old Cognac. A religious writer wrote about the redemptive value of pain as if it were in the same category as a confession.[26] I doubt whether he has ever experienced the type of pain some cancer patients endure. I look back over my personal experiences with pain and find lessons of patience and endurance, the importance of perspective, and the role of suffering in life. Anyone's allusion to the wisdom I was obtaining while I was experiencing pain would have led to my being physically or verbally abusive to him.

Suggestions

27. Don't try to convince your loved one that she can learn anything from pain—especially when it is occurring.
28. Listen without being judgmental if a loved one wants to talk about the lessons she has gained from pain.

WITNESSING PAIN

One of the most difficult things you'll ever do is hold your loved one's hand as he experiences pain, knowing you can do nothing to stop it. I served a woman with Stage IV breast cancer who was allergic to opiates. The hospice nurse tried every available painkiller. If it was effective, the allergic reactions were worse than the pain. If there weren't any allergic reactions, it was ineffectual for the pain. She knew that she would be in pain until she died. I had been volunteering for four years, and the pain of my clients was always treatable with some form of opiate. Sometimes, their pain wasn't eliminated with medication, but it became tolerable. I wasn't prepared for witnessing pain that couldn't be reduced. I visited her twice a week for a minimum of three hours each visit. We had heartfelt conversations until the pain became unbearable. When I asked her what I could do, she said, "Just hold me." The most difficult and meaningful interactions I had in hospice were holding her in my arms as waves of pain descended. I knew the only thing I could do was to silently witness it. Ask your loved one what he needs from you when the pain is uncontrollable. You might find his needs are very simple, ranging from sitting quietly next to him to playing soft music.

Suggestions

29. Hold your loved one's hand when he is experiencing pain.
30. Always ask your loved one what you can do as he experiences pain.
31. Don't feel guilty if you're not capable of witnessing intense pain.

7

EASING A LOVED ONE'S DEATH

This is the chapter you prayed wouldn't be necessary to read. You thought about the possibility of your loved one's succumbing to cancer but pushed the idea away. Now, you may fear that your hopes may be unwarranted, or worse, you know they are. Throughout my career as a speech-language pathologist, I viewed what I did as "fixing" or "helping." I worked with children and *fixed* a language problem. With adults, I *helped* stroke victims regain the ability to retrieve words and taught people who stuttered *how to use* fluency-enhancing strategies. My clients believed they were able to reengage with the world, and I believed I did something important. My roles as a "fixer" and "helper" dissolved when I became a hospice volunteer. I was told during training that every patient I would establish a relationship with, cared for, and loved would die regardless of what I did. You are now facing the same situation with your loved one. There is a Cherokee saying that "the heart is the first teacher."[1] Allow your heart to open, as threatening as it may be, as you participate in your loved one's death.

SUPPORT END-OF-LIFE DECISIONS

In most cases, people with terminal illnesses aren't choosing the "best" of all possibilities but rather the "least worst." A loved one's decision to choose death with dignity rather than add a few additional months of life with debilitating side effects may be difficult to accept. The argument goes like this: "Life is better than death, and we can spend your last months together rejoicing in the life we had. Why do you want to shorten our time together?" Be supportive of her decision even if you disagree. It may be hard to accept that your loved one is choosing to die rather than remain with you. Your acceptance of her decision to stop life-prolonging treatment is only the first step in your support. Your journey will involve caregiving issues, pain management, and hospice. You will rejoice with her about her life, become remorseful regarding a lack of accomplishments, downplay unskillful acts, and share profound insights about life and death. It's never easy saying good-bye to a friend or loved one. But supporting her nonjudgmentally will be a compassionate gift.

The decision not to extend one's life isn't straightforward. Your loved one may decide to stop life-extending treatment because the side effects aren't worth a few extra months of life. One form the decision can take is entering a hospice or contracting for home hospice services where life-extending treatments are stopped and medication is given to control pain or treat nonterminal problems (e.g., stomach virus, cold, broken bone). Hospice services are available in freestanding facilities, hospice units in hospitals, care facilities, and homes. Your loved one is eligible for hospice if a physician certifies that she has less than six months to live, and she (and sometimes you) signs a document stating that she (and you) understands that medication is given only for problems not related to extending life. Recertification is possible every six months. In eight years of hospice volunteering, I never was aware of anyone having been "kicked out" of hospice after six months. Recertification is almost automatic.

During the last stage of cancer, physicians can offer terminal sedation. Terminal sedation is defined as "the use of a sedative medication to reduce patient awareness of distressing and intractable symptoms that are insufficiently controlled by symptom-specific therapies."[2] It isn't considered a medical option until late in the cancer journey. Terminal sedation is often confused with patient-assisted suicide. They are different procedures, using different drugs, with different outcomes. Research has shown that terminal sedation does not hasten death but rather renders a person unconscious until the disease runs its course.[3] If your wife isn't responsive and you have her medical power of attorney, it's a heart-wrenching decision you may face. A patient with ALS was assigned to me. He understood the progression of his disease and knew there would be no pain involved. Despite having a caring wife and three young children, he chose terminal sedation. His wife thought it was a selfish decision. He knew his motor control would decline, leaving him with the ability to move only his eyes until the disease would stop the involuntary muscles that control respiration. The image of losing all control over the next six months was unbearable to him. Many physicians accept the use of terminal sedation for physical discomfort, but its use for psychological discomfort is controversial.[4]

Patient-assisted suicide is gaining popularity but is still controversial. Proponents who refer to it as "death with dignity" maintain that people should have the right to determine when they die. People who oppose it do so for various reasons. Religious groups don't believe we have the right to end something not our own—a God-given life. Some physicians believe that involving them in ending a life is contrary to their training. A few disability rights groups believe that it could be the first step in euthanasia for the disabled. As of January 2016, six states allow patient-assisted suicide: California, Montana, New Mexico, Washington, Vermont, and Oregon. I would encourage you to check the current status of your state's law if it's not on the above list since the death with dignity movement is gaining national support.

Hospice, terminal sedation, and patient-assisted suicide involve decisions you should discuss with your loved one long before they are necessary. A benchmark of when to begin the discussion is when your loved one receives a terminal prognosis. I have discussed each of these options with my wife and two adult children although my cancer has been stable for the past thirteen years. It wasn't a pleasant conversation, but by expressing my wishes and writing them into my last wishes document, I've taken the responsibility for my determining the end of my life out of their hands.

Suggestions

1. Support your loved one's decision to stop life-extending treatment even if you disagree.
2. Supporting your loved one's decision to stop life-extending treatment is only the first step in your support.
3. The reasons for stopping life-extending treatment can be based either on physical or psychological suffering.

SUPPORT UNREALISTIC BELIEFS
WHEN IT'S COMPASSIONATE

Everyone confronts dying differently. Compassion when a loved one faces death may require supporting unrealistic beliefs regardless of your opinion. Eventually, her views may become more realistic, but if she clings to the conviction that she will survive, accept her belief even if you are sure it's a delusion. Sometimes it's more compassionate to be complicit in a delusion rather than to crush her hope, as it was with my mother's best friend. My mother was part of a group of women whose social life revolved around shared activities and interests. All were in their sixties, and some had lost their husbands. My mother's friend had been clear with everyone for years that she feared death, and she made them promise they wouldn't tell her if she had a terminal disease. The "promise" became a running joke at their weekly mahjong games until everyone noticed their friend appeared ill. She wouldn't admit anything was wrong, but my mother learned from the woman's sister that she had terminal stomach cancer.

Despite her rapid weight loss and becoming bedridden, she refused to believe she was dying. Her friends faced a moral dilemma: Should they discuss dying with their friend of thirty years, hoping the discussion would reduce her fears, or should they honor her request and hope the unfinished aspects of their friend's life wouldn't make dying too difficult? Everyone concluded that trying to convince her she was dying would be as cruel as attempting to change her long-held beliefs. They opted for compassion, taking turns sitting at her bedside and easing her death by accepting what was important to her—a denial of her cancer.

Suggestions

4. It's more compassionate to be complicit in a delusion rather than to crush a person's hope, even if you think her beliefs are unrealistic.
5. Your nonconfrontive position may lead to your loved one's accepting her terminal condition.

WHEN TO BEGIN DISCUSSING HOSPICE

At a workshop I gave for hospice volunteers, a person who was a bedside volunteer shocked me. He admitted that he had discussed hospice with his mother only two weeks before she died, despite knowing of her terminal prognosis for three months. The Pennsylvania hospice had a quality volunteer training program emphasizing the importance of early admittance. "Why did you wait so long?" I asked. "If I had talked about hospice sooner, she would have known she was dying." I wondered what goes through the minds of people who don't understand the benefits of hospice when someone familiar with it allowed his fears to interfere with providing early compassionate services for his mother. The fear of not wanting a loved one to know she is dying contributes to the underutilization of hospice services.[5] It's a cultural problem, not one of access or knowledge. We often allow our fear of death to get in the way of helping a loved one ease into his passing. I use two criteria for determining when to begin the discussion of hospice. The first is when a loved one hears of a terminal prognosis, and the second is when he is ready to accept death.

Suggestions

6. Become knowledgeable about hospice services as soon as possible.
7. Begin exploring hospice immediately after the terminal prognosis if your loved one will accept it.
8. Don't start the discussion of hospice if your loved one does not accept the terminal diagnosis. Wait until she initiates the conversation.
9. Visit freestanding hospices and organizations providing in-home services with your loved one.

HELP YOUR LOVED ONE LET GO

"Letting go" is an ancient Buddhist concept that provides a framework for accepting those things your loved one can't control, such as extending life indefinitely.[6] All of us are born, and all of us live and *always* die. Regardless of wishes to preserve your loved one's life, you can't. Once you let go of the belief that you can change the inevitable, you'll be able to help her let go. Following is a wonderful story about letting go that involves two monks who lived in the Middle Ages in Europe.

> They vowed in their youth to abstain from sex and even forgo verbal contact with women. Both were asked to assume new assignments at a monastery some distance from their present one. The journey would be long, and being winter, they had to cross a fast-moving stream, swollen by a continuous rain. When they arrived at the stream, a beautiful young woman was standing on the bank. The older monk avoided looking at her, but the younger one turned to her with a smile and bowed. She returned his greeting.
>
> "Kindly monks, I have been standing here for three days unable to cross this raging river. I am tired, cold, and wet. Will you help me cross?"
>
> The older monk said nothing. Ignoring her, he lifted his robe and gathering it around his thighs, entered the cold water. The younger monk, still on the shore, bowed his head and with a smile said, "Of course I'll help you. Hop on my back and we'll cross together."
>
> The older monk stopped in midstream and hearing what his friend offered, turned and saw the young woman climb on the monk's back. As he stepped forward trying to maintain his balance, the older monk

stood motionless, glaring at his friend for violating their sacred vow. After the three had reached the other side, the woman dismounted.

"Thank you, kind monk. Without your help, I never could have crossed."

"You're quite welcome," he said while bowing to her.

She turned left, and the two monks turned right, continuing on the path to the monastery. The older monk, too angry to speak, said nothing during the thirty-mile journey. As they approached the monastery gates many hours later, he turned to his friend.

"How could you do that?" he asked.

"Do what?" the younger monk replied.

"What? Did you forget your vows?"

"No."

"Do they mean nothing to you?"

"They mean everything to me."

"Then how can you enter through the gates of His holiest of monasteries having had contact with a female?"

The younger monk smiled and said, "I left her at the river's edge. Why do you still carry her?"

We often grasp at useless ideas developed from the past, as did the monk in this old story. The joy you and your loved one experienced spending quiet evenings in front of the fire won't return. You wife's dream of watching her grandchildren become adults will never happen. In talking about the past, an anonymous philosopher said it's like a painting drawn on water—no trace of it remains, yet we act as if it does. Living in the past will make it more difficult for your loved one to leave. He is trying to make sense of his life—what he did and won't be able to rectify or complete. The more he can stay in the present, the easier it will be for him to accept dying. Clients and patients who focus on their past or lack of a future have more difficulty with dying than patients who focus on the present. A useful strategy for moving from the past to the present is to connect the two by highlighting the positive effects your loved one's life had on other people. A discussion of her legacy will reduce the pain of not having a future. At the bedside, I witnessed an adult child telling a dying parent how important she was in his life and how important she would remain in the lives of her grandchildren and their children because of the values she taught.

Suggestions

10. Helping your loved one let go of life is dependent on your ability to let go of her.

11. Move your loved one's fixating on past lapses in judgment to the present by highlighting the positive effects her life had on you and others.
12. If your loved one expresses the loss of the future, convince her of the legacy she leaves.

EXPECT HELPLESSNESS

People who care for a loved one with terminal cancer experience profound helplessness.[7] Despite wanting to save them, they can't. Your goal is not to rescue your loved one but rather to provide emotional support and physical comfort. I started hospice knowing there would be no miracles for the patients I served. I knew every person I established a relationship with would die within six months—usually much sooner. Throughout our six-month training, this concept was emphasized. I accepted it, although I felt helpless when my first patient was dying. We had established a close relationship, and I knew I would be distraught when he died. I asked a hospice nurse how she accepted the loss of those for whom she cared. She replied,

> Love can take many forms. The love I experience for my patients involves knowing I did everything I could to make their death as peaceful as possible. I know everyone I care for will die within six months. If I focused on their death, I'd go crazy or quit. But when you know you're helping them on a journey, your love is different. So is your sense of loss. Yes, I miss most of the patients I've served, but it's minor compared to what I gave them and they gave back to me.[8]

Her wise observations became the key to dealing with my sense of helplessness. I wasn't there to rescue but rather to ease my patient's journey. I asked myself when leaving the bedside *Did I do something today that will ease my patient's death?* If I had, it was a good day for both of us. If I hadn't, I tried to determine what to do differently when I returned the following week. The same guiding maxim applies to your loved one.

Suggestion

13. Realize that your goal is not to save your loved one but to serve her as she dies.

DYING IS HARD WORK

Dying will be exhausting for you and your loved one. It's not an event but rather a process. One patient said to me "You know, dying is such hard work." For two months her physical condition declined, and I assumed she was referring to her pulmonary problems. She paused and said, "I'm not just talking about what's happening to my body." Pointing to her head, she continued, "The hard work is also happening up here." You should expect your loved one to vacillate between exhaustion from the drugs and effects of the cancer and euphoria from the temporary relief of pain. Accept both as fleeting moments and hope the euphoria will last until she dies, but know that it never does. We hope the exhaustion lasts only a short time, but experience tells us it's unlikely. Families of patients often become jubilant when many of the end-of-life behaviors abate or disappear. They hope the medical community was wrong and that they are witnessing a miracle. While both are possible, it's rare. Relish your loved one's euphoria as a short, peaceful moment in time. Dying is a time of great emotional turmoil. One that moves through all time frames. Regrets over what was or wasn't done live in the past. Hope, such as wishing the pain will stop or the euphoria will last until a loved one dies, is thrust into the future. As much as possible, remain in the present. Accept what your loved one is enduring as part of the cancer journey.

Suggestions

14. Approach dying as a process rather than as an event with clear beginning and end points.
15. Expect long-term exhaustion and short-lived euphoria.
16. The hard work of dying involves both the body and the mind.

DON'T BE AFRAID TO TALK ABOUT DEATH

There is a Tibetan saying that goes "Tomorrow or the next life—which comes first, we never know."[9] Unlike the Tibetans we avoid talking about death, especially with our loved one. Your hesitancy may be based on the belief that your loved one doesn't want to talk about her death. Don't be afraid of selecting words you believe may be inappropriate. You'll say the right ones if they come from the heart and are tempered by your head.

Producing the "right" words has much in common with what happens in music. I struggled to produce the "right" notes in a traditional song I was learning when I first started playing the Shakuhachi. My teacher, who is a great musician and wise philosopher, said, "Stop worrying about the notes. Think how you would play the song to your son when he was a baby." For my teacher, notes came from one's soul, not from the flute. The same applies in deciding what to say to your loved one or friend about her passing.

I served a man in hospice who knew he was dying from testicular cancer, as did his wife. They prided themselves on thirty years of honesty and openness and conversing about everything, ranging from the latest Giants baseball results to congressional ethics. But during the two months I visited them in their home, she never once used the words "dying," "death," or "passing" or talked about her husband's deteriorating condition. He wanted to talk about his death to only me. I asked whether he had ever discussed these issues with his wife. "No," he said. "It would upset her." She confided in me when we were alone that although she wanted to talk about end-of-life issues with her husband, she was afraid it would upset him. I suggested to each one individually that it might be time for the conversation each believed the other didn't want to begin. The fear of using emotionally laden words prevented this couple from speaking about important issues until it was almost too late.

In eight years as a bedside hospice volunteer, I never once initiated a discussion about death with my patients. Almost all of them eventually wanted to talk about it, approaching end-of-life discussions either obliquely (e.g., I guess I should update my will) or directly (e.g., I'm afraid of dying). Listen nonjudgmentally, answer with facts, and don't be afraid to ask your loved one whether he would like a visit from a counselor or spiritual adviser. Many people believe that as someone approaches death, his need to communicate diminishes, based on the reduced verbal output from people who are dying. Actually, the reverse is true.[10] We misperceive a reduction in words as a decrease in need. People who are dying are facing the most difficult transition they will ever encounter. Everything about them is changing. Silence in the dying is less a sign of not wishing to communicate and more a sign of uncertainty, fear, or regret.

Many great thinkers have said that everything appears difficult until you know how to do it. The same is also true about talking of death. In discussing it with your loved one, don't be surprised if the discomfort takes the form of resistance or silence, as it did for a man diagnosed with schizophrenia and terminal lung cancer. He was found in a filthy one-room

apartment in San Francisco's Tenderloin District and sent to a hospice facility operated by the Sisters of Charity, Mother Teresa's religious order.
Most of the patients sat in the garden area every day, socialized, smoked,
and reminisced. Some patients had received a compassionate release from
state prisons and talked about their wasted lives. My patient never left his
room despite being capable. He was curled up in bed close to the wall
when I entered his room. "Hi, Harry, can I sit with you for a while?" He
glanced in my direction, nodded, and turned back to the wall. I sat next
to him for the next forty minutes, and he occasionally glanced at me. After
forty minutes of silence, I said, "Harry, I have to go now. Thank you for
letting me visit with you. Would you like me to come back next week?"
I expected him to either remain silent or say no. "Yes," he said, without
any hesitation, "I'd like that a lot." Our second meeting began as had the
first. After about fifteen minutes of silence, he said, "I'm afraid of dying. Do
you know what it's like?" I proceeded to tell him what I had experienced
with the deaths of other people. We talked for over thirty minutes, and he
initiated the topics of his concern. There was nothing psychotic about his
words or behaviors. His fears were similar to the most articulate insights of
people I served. At our third meeting, he asked me to set up a small model
train set. It was his most prized possession, one of the few things he had
brought to the hospice. As I changed the direction of the tracks and rearranged the cars, he kept asking questions about dying. *Will there be pain?
What happens after I die? Where will my body go?* I returned for our fourth
meeting and found the train set and an empty bed.

Suggestions

17. Don't spend time searching for the right words. Speak from your
    heart and you'll be fine.
18. Don't initiate a conversation about dying if your loved one isn't
    ready. Wait until she initiates it.
19. Allow periods of silence to be the preparation your loved one
    needs to talk about his death.

DON'T ASSUME SPIRITUALITY
AND RELIGION ARE ENOUGH

In my eight years as a hospice volunteer, I never saw two people approach
their death in the same way. Some people did it without spirituality, and

others relied on it and their religion. There was also a vast difference within each group. Many of the differences had to do with their personal history. Some people viewed cancer within a religious context, a test from God or a malady they could overcome with the Deity's blessings. Others saw cancer as a way of learning something about themselves. The relationship of illness to a supreme being also was viewed as a betrayal by God. A client said to me, "If He is so powerful, why couldn't He prevent this from happening to me? I worshipped Him my entire life, and this is how He repays me?" Some people who had never been religious grabbed on to any set of beliefs that gave them hope, from becoming a born-again Baptist to embracing a Buddhist belief in reincarnation.

The mother of a woman I served in hospice filled her daughter's room every day with more than thirty votive candles, each with a picture of a saint. She believed that if her faith were strong enough, her daughter would live despite having terminal pharyngeal cancer. Clutching her beliefs became painful for the mother. I have found that the greater the religious conviction, the greater people's expectations are that a loved one's condition will improve. The daughter's convictions were at best moderate. She believed that her mother's incessant prayers had more to do with the mother's inability to face life without her daughter than anything else. Despite a readiness to die, the daughter held on to life until she believed her mother could live without her. The mother, who had been religious her entire life, felt God had abandoned her. She confided to the hospice staff after her daughter had died that this was the first time she had asked God to intervene and he hadn't. God's allowing her daughter to die had crushed her faith.

Audiences at book readings and presentations often ask me whether people who believe in an afterlife or reincarnation find it easier to die than those who don't have religious or spiritual beliefs. I think most people expected to hear that there was a direct and positive connection between faith or spirituality and the acceptance of death. A belief in a supreme being for many people did ease their death. But for others, equally religious, completing unresolved issues was more important. For example, a devout client didn't believe God could forgive his "sins" for something horrendous he did as a teenager. "What I did was so terrible that if he were alive, he couldn't forgive me and I can't forgive myself." A person who receives a terminal diagnosis or believes the cancer will end his life may look for assurances that something exists beyond what he knows. I served a Presbyterian minister who invited his congregation to visit him in the hospice for prayer sessions. The purpose wasn't to ask for a miracle cure but rather to help him prepare for death. Conversely, a devoutly religious Catholic woman who feared death prayed every day for a miracle. A man with no religious beliefs was comfortable preparing for his death because he had taken care of all unfinished business. "No matter what's beyond," he said, "I'm going there with a clean plate."

Your friend's tolerance of your religious beliefs before she became ill may have changed, as it did with a person who was a lifelong atheist. Her aunt, a respected member of the family, was a born-again Christian and believed that unless she could bring her niece to Jesus, she would suffer eternal damnation. Her self-imposed obligation to save her niece took the form of constant monologues asserting the importance of conversion. Her niece felt assaulted by beliefs she never could accept and frightened by visions conjured by her aunt's vivid imagination. From experience, I've found deathbed conversions are rare. Insistence that a friend convert implies that many of the things she believed throughout her life had been wrong. This is not the time to castigate a friend who is preparing to die, even if you think the outcome will bring her to God's hands. Your friend or loved one is trying to understand her life. Honor her beliefs regardless of your views of the afterlife.

Suggestions

20. Neither spirituality nor religion by itself may be enough to ease a loved one's death.
21. Regardless of your loved one's spirituality or religious convictions, search for any unfinished business that might be making the transition more difficult.
22. Don't attempt a deathbed conversion. Efforts generate more annoyance than creation of states of grace.
23. Honor your loved one's beliefs regardless of how much you believe they will result in terrible afterlife consequences.

ASKING FOR FORGIVENESS

Most of us can find something in our lives that we prefer not to have done. It can be a minor transgression such as not acknowledging the help someone provided or something unspeakable, as with my patient who believed he was responsible for the death of his son. Your response to a loved one's asking for forgiveness should be straightforward: "I forgive you." It's irrelevant whether you mean it. Your goal should be to ease your loved one's transition, not express your "true feelings." Dying is not about you. That was the theme I witnessed when I heard a physically abusive patient ask his daughter to forgive him. It was one of the most magnanimous gestures I saw in hospice. Although she said, "I forgive you, Dad," she couldn't forgive him for what he had done, but she understood that his abuse forty years ago had come from alcoholism. She told me it was one of the hardest things she had ever done.

Not all efforts to obtain forgiveness go as well as it did with the daughter who possessed a reservoir of compassion. A hospice patient had abandoned her two daughters when they were teenagers. Guilt consumed her because of what she had done. Now, as adults and knowing she was dying, her children refused to visit her or take her phone calls. It's not unusual for the person who is being asked to forgive to decline or not be reachable (e.g., died, can't be located, or someone from the distant past). Think about substitutes if that occurs. I suggested to the woman that we write a letter to be delivered to them after she had died. I didn't realize when I made the suggestion that it would be a consuming event for her. I visited her every week for three hours. For three weeks she struggled to put her emotions into words. I would read back what she had dictated and wait for her response. "No, that's not what I mean" or "I'm not using the right words" were typical responses. After a month of visits, she had me write, "I'm sorry for the hurt I caused you. Please forgive me. I always loved you." She sat back in her chair, smiled, and said, "Yes, that's it." She became calm and died peacefully a week later.

For people still alive who refuse to talk to your loved one, other intermediary methods besides letters can be used, such as leaving phone messages when the person won't speak to your loved one or sending text messages and emails. A different problem occurs when someone who doesn't need forgiveness asks for it. One client asked her adult children for forgiveness for her transgressions. Both children were confused. She had sacrificed everything for them, and in their eyes, she was a saint. The more she asked for forgiveness, the more insistent her children were that she had never done anything wrong to warrant being forgiven. It was painful to watch her ask for forgiveness and hear her children not provide it because they felt there was no need. I suggested to the children that they honor their mother's request, regardless of whether they believed there was any need for it. I explained that asking for forgiveness may involve recollections of events (correct or not) that their mother didn't wish to share. The next time she asked for forgiveness, they gave it. It appeared to everyone present in the room that a great burden had been lifted from her soul.

Suggestions

24. If your loved one asks for forgiveness, grant it, without qualifications or lengthy rebuttals.
25. Create substitute forms of forgiveness if your loved one can't be forgiven by the offended person.
26. Forgive your loved one when she asks for it, even if you don't think she did anything that requires forgiveness.

HELP TIE UP LOOSE ENDS

There is an obsession with tying up loose ends as a person comes closer to dying. Sometimes it's literal, such as asking for forgiveness, forgiving others, or balancing a bank book. But with many people, the loose ends can be an allegory. On entering a patient's room, I saw him opening drawers and rummaging through his clothes. "Jean, can I help you with anything?" Not stopping his efforts, he glanced at me and said, "It's my manuscript. I can't find it, and it's due at the publisher's tomorrow." I helped him back into bed and said, "I'll look for it. Why don't you rest?" He had been a war correspondent in World War II and credited with changing combat journalism. I proceeded to open all the drawers and closets and even looked under the bed. After searching for fifteen minutes, I said, "It's not here." It was a response that agitated him. He tried to get out of bed again, but I gently restrained him. "I know Mary will be here soon," I said. "I'm sure she knows where it is." Mary was a good friend who had a long history with him. If anybody knew where it was, it would be Mary. He laid back down and fell asleep. As soon as Mary arrived I said, "Jean was looking for his manuscript. Do you know where it is?" She looked confused. "What manuscript? He hasn't written anything in twenty years." She told me one of Jean's greatest regrets was not doing anything with his career.

As Mary and I talked, Jean awoke. "The manuscript. Did you find it?" Without any hesitation Mary said, "I'm sorry, Jean. I forgot to tell you I sent it out yesterday." Jean smiled and said, "Thank you." I never knew what the manuscript represented but both Mary and I thought it was missed opportunities. For another client, what was unfinished was even more obscure. Four days before his death, his daughter found him in the garage straightening out nut and bolt containers. "Dad, what are you doing?" she said. He responded, "The shelves are too messy." She assumed he was delirious and helped him back into his room over protests that he wasn't finished. The next day when she visited, he was again in the garage rearranging the jars. "Dad, what are you doing?" Once again he said, "The shelves are too messy. I have to clean them up." This time instead of forcing him back to bed, she said, "Let me help you." For the next ten minutes they both rearranged the items until her father was satisfied; then she again helped him to bed. We both felt that rearranging the objects was her father's way of trying to put some order into his life. His daughter had no idea what it was that he thought was unfinished, but she said that after they had completed the task, he became calm.

If your loved one insists on doing something such as finding a lost object or rearranging things, don't argue. Just help. If you can identify what remains unfinished, try to help him complete it. If the activity has nothing to do with his life, assume that it's an allegory, but treat it as if it's the actual unfinished activity.

Suggestions

27. Don't dismiss the need for completing unfinished business.
28. Some efforts to "clean one's plate" before dying are literal, while others are allegorical.
29. Participate in any attempts that seem related to finishing something.

SAYING AND ACCEPTING THANKS

We are often reluctant to thank the person who is dying for all she has done and what she means to us. Many people believe that by thanking a dying person, they are confirming her imminent death. Long before friends and loved ones express their gratitude, her body has told her that she is dying. By thanking your loved one, you are saying she made a difference in your life. My friend who had previously told me she had cancer called when she was in hospice and had only a few days to live. She thanked me, using simple and honest words, for being her friend. It was one of the most humbling conversations I have ever had. Your loved one may need to thank you for contributions to his life. Gratitude from someone who knows he is dying is heartfelt. Accept it with graciousness. Don't minimize the thanks given to you for making his life meaningful. Few people are comfortable with end-of-life conversations. One way of reducing the discomfort is to host a good-bye party. I had the honor of attending three when I was a hospice volunteer. The one for a local San Francisco actor was the most joyful. When I first met Dean in his apartment, he showed me the chair Tennessee Williams had sat in when they discussed the state of theater in San Francisco. "We were good friends," he said. "Well, maybe not friends, but colleagues. I'm sure if he were still alive he would be at my good-bye party." He told me about an elaborate affair that his friends and the actors he had helped were organizing. "Why should they celebrate my life when I'm not there?" he asked. The planning had started when he had received a terminal prognosis. The choreography had to be worthy of opening night on Broadway since Dean had been an actor for sixty years. "And, of course, I expect you to be there."

One week later, as instructed, I entered the lobby of a theater where he often performed. He entered the room through an elevator in a Shakespearian gown appropriate for King Lear. He began reciting lines from a play as he was wheeled out into the room. The applause was thunderous. "Thank you all for coming," Dean said when the applause stopped. "Now, it's time to celebrate." Overflowing trays of food and many glasses of expensive champagne came out of the kitchen. His closest friends went to his side and told him how much he meant to them and how he had contributed to their lives. Most were local actors, but a few I recognized from films and television. Many wept throughout their conversations with Dean. They expressed gratitude for having been allowed into the life of this wonderful person. He often recounted the party's events during the time I served him, marveling how it was the culmination of his life. The following was reported in the local newspaper after he died:

> Mr. Goodman requested that there be no memorial service, but a celebration of his life was held at ACT on June 19. The evening, attended by Mr. Goodman and some 200 guests, included a reading of his newest play, "Bloody August." At the ceremony, Mr. Goodman received a special lifetime achievement award from Actors' Equity for 63 years of service to the union and to the theater.[11]

Following Dean's death, I knew what I wanted on my headstone: "He made a difference." That should become a guiding principle for a good-bye party as well as for shepherding your loved one to her death—the belief that she made a difference. It doesn't require worldwide implications. Rather, it can be as simple as her understanding that the values she inculcated in family and friends will create a legacy that will transcend her life. When my brother-in-law was still alert, I would read emails from people whose lives he affected for fifty years. Just before he began actively dying, we invited friends to call in their thanks. Some of the phone calls my brother-in-law listened to as they occurred. Others were played back to him on the answering machine.

Often, people may be uncomfortable thanking a person for all she contributed to their lives and accepting her gratitude. A public display of affection and thankfulness makes it easier for those wanting to testify to a person's contributions. At another good-bye party, a local poet handed each person a sheet of paper with one poem written on it as they came to her side. After the last guest had received his poem, she said, "Now, I'm ready to die." The party allowed friends to thank her for being in their life, and it gave her an opportunity to thank them with her most precious items—her poems. It's a blessing for your loved one to have a roomful of friends and family offer thanks and chronicle a lifetime of her achievements. Ask your loved one to be involved in the planning. Memories of the event will last you a lifetime.

Suggestions

30. Help your loved one complete unfinished tasks.
31. Accept all expressions of gratitude even if you think that what you did was inconsequential.
32. Host a good-bye party.
33. Encourage your loved one's family and friends to publically express thanks for all she contributed to them.

DON'T GRIEVE EXCESSIVELY IN YOUR LOVED ONE'S PRESENCE

There is a difference between grieving the eventual loss of a person and demonstrating it in her presence. Excessive emotional displays can be detrimental to a more peaceful death. One of my hospice patients was a woman in her fifties who was dying of lung cancer. Her father was at her side and so distraught that he often couldn't speak. When he left the room, the daughter asked, "How will he live without me?" She vowed to remain alive, despite the intense pain she was experiencing, until her father could accept her death. The father's grief, while a display of his needs, prolonged his daughter's death. To grieve is natural and a way in which we demonstrate our connection with the world. Grief can serve many functions, some intended and some not. I was at a bedside when friends and relatives believed it was all right to express their grief since their loved one was in a coma. What they didn't realize is that hearing is thought to be one of the last senses to shut down before death.[12] Even if your loved one appears un-responsive, assume that she can hear your words and intonation. For your loved one's sake, if your grief becomes uncontrollable, leave her room and return when you're composed. Not displaying grief shouldn't be confused with the concept of "keeping a still upper lip." Rather, it's placing the needs of your loved one over your own.

Suggestions

34. The excessive display of grief in front of your loved one can pro-long her dying.
35. Assume that your loved one can hear you even if she is in a coma since hearing is one of the last senses to leave.

DON'T FORCE FOOD OR WATER

The body no longer requires nourishment or liquid when it is shutting down.[13] The distressful behaviors exhibited by the person beginning active dying do not come from hunger or thirst. The natural reaction to an ill person with no appetite is to suggest they eat or drink "to keep up their strength." The ingestion of either food or liquids near the end of life can be painful. Accept your loved one's decision to stop eating or drinking, since the loss of appetite is an indication she is having difficulty processing food and fluid. The decision to stop eating and drinking doesn't always mean death will occur soon. The disease, not a lack of nutrition, will cause death.

Sometimes cultural practices can be detrimental to an easier death. A Vietnamese grandfather whose teenage grandson was dying kept forcing him to eat despite the hospice staff's warning that it was painful. He would hide food and give it to his grandson when staff members weren't present. Our patient, who was a dutiful grandson, consumed whatever the grandfa-ther insisted he eat. The staff would realize that the grandfather had again snuck in food only when the grandson would experience pain followed by explosive vomiting. The hospice team faced a moral dilemma. Their first obligation was to the patient, but barring the grandfather from being at his grandson's side would have been devastating to the family. An interpreter was called in to unravel the problem. The grandfather, according to the interpreter, feared that his grandson would become a "hungry ghost" if he didn't eat before dying. A hungry ghost is a mythological figure with an insatiable appetite who roams the earth with a mouth so small that he can't ingest food or water.[14] According to the grandfather, if his grandson left this life hungry or thirsty, he would become a hungry ghost. Only after a Buddhist spiritual counselor explained to the grandfather that his interpretation of hungry ghosts was wrong did he stop sneaking food and drink to his grandson.

Suggestions

36. Don't force your loved one to ingest either food or liquids if her body is shutting down.
37. Don't expect death to occur soon after food and fluids are stopped.
38. Use a sponge paddle to alleviate dryness in the mouth or on the lips.

GIVE LEGITIMACY TO PRIVATE EXPERIENCES

People who are dying may encounter visions or sounds visible or audible only to them.[15] Give legitimacy to these visions, whether you believe they're real or the result of changes in the brain's chemistry. Don't try to interpret, and don't insist the vision isn't real unless it's disturbing to your loved one. If the vision is disturbing, don't rely just on words to reduce his anxiety but also refer to objects he can see. My brother-in-law mistook the side rails on his bed for the bars in a jail cell. My wife and I were in Hawaii, and he was on the East Coast. My attempts to convince him over the phone that he couldn't be in jail didn't work. I tried to think of another strategy. I asked him to look at the wall and tell me what he saw. "Mom's painting," he said. "Where is it hanging?" I asked. "In my apartment," he replied. "Where are you if it's hanging on your apartment wall and you see it? He thought for a moment before saying, "I guess I'm in my apartment." I responded, "Then you can't be in jail, right? Without hesitation, he said, "Of course not!" It was the key to relieving his anxiety and a strategy I relied on whenever the visions were frightening.

Most visions are pleasant, as they were for a patient who told me he saw his wife, who had died ten years earlier, at the end of his bed. He had spoken about her often, their life together and the terrible pain he had experienced since she had died ten years ago. "You think I'm crazy, don't you?" he said. "No," I replied. "Many of my patients say they see someone from their past who is no longer alive." He responded, "And you believe them?" I said, "What they see is real to them, and that's what matters." He proceeded to tell me about their life together and how her calm presence at the foot of his bed made him less concerned about dying. He often spoke about his life during my visits. I don't think he would have shared the events of his fulfilling life with me if I had dismissed his encounter with his deceased wife.

Suggestions

39. Accept your loved one's private experiences if they are uplifting.
40. Don't interpret uplifting private experiences.
41. Help your loved one dismiss frightening visions through objective means rather than words.

GIVE PERMISSION TO DIE

Your final gift to your loved one is giving her permission to die. Use simple words coupled with how important she was in your life. Giving permission to die should be combined with endearing words that proclaim the positive effects your loved one had on your life. Use simple words such as "I know how hard you're holding on, Mom, but it's all right to let go now. I love you and will miss you; you have made a difference in my life." Other people at the bedside should express similar thoughts, but permission to die should be granted only once unless you think your loved one didn't comprehend your words. If other people are at the bedside, each one should echo your thoughts. Also, rarely does granting permission to die immediately result in someone's death. Letting go of life can take days.

The timing of death is still a mystery to me. I've witnessed people struggling to maintain their life force regardless of how accepting I thought they were of death. This "scheduling" leads me to believe loved ones who are dying may control the moment of death more than we can understand, holding on to life until they feel that those they care about are ready for them to depart. The ability to schedule one's death was apparent with my brother-in-law. My wife and daughter left for the East Coast when it was apparent he was close to dying. My son and I were to leave in a few days from San Francisco. My wife called after having arrived and said she thought my brother-in-law was actively dying. Listening to all the changes that had happened since their last visit, I knew she was right. I asked my daughter to place the phone receiver next to his ear, although according to my daughter he was no longer responsive. In an earlier conversation, I had told him I would help him die. When I reiterated the promise over the phone, my daughter said tears flowed from the corner of one of his eyes. Ten hours passed before my son and I were able to join them. As the taxi drove us to his apartment, I was sure he was no longer alive. "He's been waiting for you," my daughter said when we entered the apartment. Within two hours after I had arrived and fulfilled my promise, he peacefully died.

How often have you heard of someone feeling guilty because during the few minutes she was gone from the room, her loved one died? I believe some people who are actively dying want to spare loved ones from witnessing their death and choose to die when they're not present. The decision to die when a person leaves the room is more about a loved one's concern than anything negative in their relationship. In all the years that I served people who were dying, I could never determine why some people chose to die during those few moments a loved one left the room, but I believe it comes from love.

Suggestions

42. Your final gift to your loved one will be permission to die.
43. Use simple words and state the offer only once or, if you believe your loved one didn't comprehend what you said, a few times more.
44. Loved ones may be able to "schedule" their death.
45. Your loved one's dying when you leave the room is more an act of love than a statement of anything negative about your relationship.

HOW TO CREATE A VIGIL

A vigil is a procedure where you or a hospice vigil volunteer remove everything associated with your loved one's disease. Of course, some necessary palliative care items will remain (e.g., oxygen tank, urine bag, etc.), but items such as medicine, bed pads, or absorbent briefs should be placed out of your loved one's line of vision. Surround him with objects, smells, sounds, and people important to him. You may experience discomfort when you are alone with your loved one when he begins actively dying, or when managing the interactions of friends and relatives who gather. Let the volunteer structure and manage the setting. She can come into your home or care facility, guide those who aren't sure of what to do, help create a calming environment, offer suggestions for easing the death of your loved one, and if necessary manage friends and relatives.

I was asked to create a vigil for a patient whose partner was uncomfortable being alone with him as he died. Together, we rearranged the room. Pictures of him in his youth surrounded by members of his motorcycle club filled the room along with motorcycle memorabilia. I brought a CD of songs that he had said took him to a place I couldn't follow, and his partner surrounded his bed with bouquets of his favorite flowers. It was a marvelous death. Conversely, the most disruptive death I witnessed was when two daughters who had bickered their entire lives carried their hostility into their mother's vigil. I asked both of them to join me outside of their mother's room, and I explained the effects their arguing had on their mother. Although both believed I was meddling in their affairs, the bickering stopped when they reentered their mother's room. The vigil serves two purposes if it is done right, as it was with my motorcycle patient. The first is to create a positive environment in which you ease a loved one's passing. The second is to create endearing memories for friends and loved ones to retain.

Suggestions

46. Remove objects associated with the disease or its treatment.
47. Fill the room with objects, music, and smells having a positive connection with your loved one's life.
48. Ask the hospice volunteer to be responsible for the vigil if you are uncomfortable managing it.
49. A vigil will ease your loved one's death and create positive memories for you.

WHAT TO DO WHEN DEATH IS IMMINENT

Many poets and authors try to describe the sensations they experienced at the moment of someone's death. I have been present many times, but I still can't find adequate words to describe it. People speak about a sense of spirituality pervading the room, a heightened sense of awareness, the flood of memories surfacing, and indescribable love for the person who is leaving.[16] Nobody ever spoke about anything frightening; people describe the actual moment of death as moving and always peaceful. Four of us were present at the passing of a patient to whom we were close. Each of us had different spiritual convictions, ranging from religious to agnostic. In conversations we had after our patient's death, we were surprised that what we experienced was similar.

Rely on a loved one's history to ease her journey. Don't worry about doing the "right" thing. Rather, focus on listening and observing. Your words and actions will be compassionate and helpful if your heart is open. Your loved one's history can provide you with guidelines for easing her death. For example, a loved one who never wanted to be touched may be uncomfortable with someone holding her hand or touching her body as she dies. Conversely, a history of a loved one's need to touch or be touched suggests that you should hold his hand or touch his body. Just before my brother-in-law died, my wife laid next to him and cradled him as if he were a sleeping child. It was an experience that she remembers eight years after his death, and one that still provides comfort. You will instinctually know what to do if you let the situation instruct you. Don't worry about doing the "right" thing; just listen and watch. If your heart is open, your words and actions will be compassionate and helpful.

Suggestions

50. No words can describe what you will feel at the death of your loved one.
51. Listen to and observe what is happening to your loved one before you act.
52. Rely on your loved one's history to find words and behaviors to ease her death.

WHAT TO DO AFTER THE MOMENT OF DEATH

Sit and do nothing. Don't call the hospice or the mortician until you are ready to say good-bye. This is a time to reflect on what your loved one's life and death mean to you. A ritual commemorating her life and your relationship is appropriate. It can serve two important functions. The first is to connect you to memories of your life with her. The ritual can involve traditional behaviors such as an act of kneeling for Catholics, touching one's head to the ground for Muslims, and an offering of gratitude for Buddhists. These rituals have a religious basis, but others are secular. I improvised a piece on my Shakuhachi when I was in a hospice following the death of each patient I had served. What I played was spontaneous and a way of expressing my love. I felt the notes were inspired, but I couldn't remember what I had played when I left the room. The second function of a ritual is to honor your friend's life. A client celebrated the passing of her partner through a traditional Irish wake. She surrounded her with flowers, incense, and pictures of their life together. Everyone remembered the wonderful times they all had. The stories told were irreverent, raunchy, and humorous.

Her friends and partner looked back on the memories they created and felt fortunate they knew such an incredible person.

Many people find it healing to clean a loved one's body in preparation for removal. I asked my wife, son, and daughter and my brother-in-law's favorite professional caregiver if they wished to participate in cleaning his body and preparing him for the mortician. Everyone agreed, but I could tell there was some discomfort. No one had done this before other than me, and my experience was with only one patient. Their discomfort changed as we removed his bedclothes and washed his body with warm, scented water. My wife focused on cleaning his face as everyone else washed his body. Through touching stories, each of us spoke about his impact on our lives. We included him in conversations although we knew he couldn't respond. After we had cleaned his body, we dressed him in his favorite T-shirt and shorts. It's been eight years since his death, and the image of my brother-in-law lying in bed wearing his favorite clothes still provides lasting memories. Don't be afraid to invent a ritual. The manner of preparation and the care taken will develop permanent touchstones for reducing your grief.

Suggestions

53. Sit and do nothing.
54. Reflect on your loved one's life and the impact she had on you.
55. Create a ritual.
56. Ceremoniously clean and prepare your loved one's body.

YOU DID THE BEST YOU COULD

We rarely act in a vacuum. What we do and say are often the result of our history and events swirling around us. We do the best we can within a world whose demands often outpace our capabilities. One of the most challenging, transformative, and rewarding things you will ever do is provide compassionate care near the end of your loved one's life. I have spoken with numerous people who've chastised themselves for "not doing a better job" for their loved one or friend. One person told me about having to decide whether to allow her father to die or remain on life support. He had given her his medical power of attorney. The monitors indicated there was no brain activity, and the medical staff asked her to decide when to withdraw life support. Her father's sister wanted him to remain on it indefinitely. The daughter wrestled with the decision for two days. She disregarded the sister's wishes and told the medical staff to remove all life-sustaining medical devices. Two years after his death, she still wondered whether she had been too hasty in having the life-sustaining devices removed, asking herself whether she should have preserved his life for a few more days or weeks, hoping there would be some sign of brain activity.

We all have questioned whether we did the right thing at certain times in our life. Years ago when my life was in turmoil, I spent a weekend at the Shasta Abbey Buddhist Monastery. I raised my hand when the abbot asked whether anyone wished to receive counseling. The next day I entered the room and saw a monk who was in his twenties—no more than half my age at the time. My reluctance to share my problems with him faded after a few minutes, and I forgot that he had no experience with marriage or children and most likely had just begun shaving. I spoke about the unskillful things I had done as a father and a husband. After about twenty minutes I stopped. He remained motionless for a few minutes before saying, "Stan, we do the best we can, given the circumstances of our lives." He rose and left the room. It took me a while to understand the importance of his words. What we do and say are often products of what precedes our actions and events swirling around us, many of which we have no control over.

Suggestions

57. The demands on you may be greater than your ability to fulfill them.
58. You did the best you could given the circumstances of your life.

LESSONS YOU WILL LEARN

You may find the idea of learning anything from the death of your loved one macabre, but the lessons are profound and rarely come from more mundane experiences. During my first four years of hospice, I realized that I was receiving lessons from my patients during every visit. They started on my first shift when I was caring for a patient with infectious hepatitis who had little bowel control and was incontinent. The twelve hours I was with him were filled with challenges to my greatest fears. The lessons I learned were only the first of hundreds to come. The meaning of many of them was immediately evident, such as the importance of offering thanks. But other lessons, such as realizing the relationship between understanding and compassion, took time to comprehend. Instead of trying to determine their significance, I wrote what I witnessed during each visit. At the end of four years, I had more than five hundred pages of observations and stories. A shortened version of my

notes became my memoir, *Lessons for the Living: Stories of Forgiveness, Gratitude, and Courage at the End of Life*.[17] I still struggle to understand some of the
lessons, and others have been guiding my life for years. From the death of my
mother, I began to understand the importance of telling people how important they are in my life. My brother-in-law's death taught me the importance
of leading a meaningful life. The death of a good friend showed me that it
was possible to accept the inevitable while embracing every second of life. I
learned the importance of forgiveness from an ex-heroin addict whose family
was delighted that he was dying; the power of compassion from watching an
elderly and angry woman change her life one month before she died in my
arms; the need for friendship from the founder of a historic collection of gay
erotic art who was afraid that he would die alone; selflessness from a teenager
suffering from cystic fibrosis who was more concerned about the distress
he was causing his mother than the pain he experienced with each breath;
and living in the present from a woman who, while holding her infant and
knowing he would be dead within a few days, thanked friends and family for
a surprise Mother's Day party.

These individuals and others have provided lessons so meaningful that
they grabbed me and said, "Listen, this is important." I did, and they changed
my life. These and many other lessons took time for me to understand. If
anyone had suggested that these were "learning" events when they were occurring, I'm not sure what I would have said, but I doubt the words would
have been pleasant. So in advance, I offer apologies for suggesting that anything teachable will come from the death of your loved one. Six months
from now, come back to this section and reread it. The Buddha said that just
as an elephant leaves the biggest footprint in the jungle, so does death when
it comes to living.[18] You will have the greatest opportunity to learn how to
live when you are in the presence of a loved one who will soon die. In the
Middle Ages, spiritual leaders and scholars of the Catholic Church wrote a
"manual for dying" called the *Book of the Craft of Dying*, or *Ars Moriendi*.[19]
The text provides instructions for creating a good death. Some say the most
important lesson is "learn how to die and you'll learn how to live."

Suggestions

59. You will receive gems of wisdom from participating in a loved
    one's death.
60. Don't try to understand the lessons when they are occurring. It
    may take months or even years for you to appreciate them.

8

RECOVERING JOY

You have lost a loved one, a key person in your life, and without her, nothing matters anymore. The pain is so intense that you question whether you'll ever risk developing another meaningful relationship if the price is feeling what you are now experiencing. The cost for recovering joy is the willingness to experience pain. You can insulate yourself from pain, but in the process, you will stop engaging. An unwillingness to again lose something that makes your life meaningful can result in a decision to disengage from the world. Your grief is so great it echoes the pain expressed by Henry IV in Shakespeare's *History of Richard II.*[1]

> My grief lies all within;
> And these external manners of laments
> Are merely shadows of the unseen grief
> That swells with silence in the tortured soul.

Richard II spoke of a pain so intense that any external expression could not match what he felt. What Shakespeare didn't address was how one reengages when life turns meaningless. One strategy is to view life as if it were a dance. Think of the tango with its twists, turns, dips, and wild spins. Those who sit and watch can never experience the dancer's joy. Yes, the dancers may risk embarrassment by fumbling over their feet or bumping into each other as they learn new routines. You watch them, and at times they are so in sync with the music that you cannot imagine one without the other. You can experience life only if you choose to go out on the dance floor and not remain a spectator. In this chapter, you'll learn how to tango.

UNDERSTANDING GRIEF'S INTENSITY

There are no hierarchies when it comes to losses. Grieving the loss of social contacts is no less important than mourning the loss of intimacy. Grief is grief regardless of its origin. Its intensity is related to how integral the loss is to your identity. The greater the identification or dependence, the greater the grief. A caregiver whom I counseled was distraught after her husband of forty-five years died after battling cancer for ten years. She restructured her life during that time to care for her husband, giving up a position with the potential to produce an exciting career. She didn't resent her husband but rather did everything for him from a profound sense of love and loyalty. Friends assumed that she would experience relief following his death since she was his primary caregiver and everything she did had to factor in her husband's needs. Her friends were shocked when she became despondent after his death. Yes, it was good that she was no longer responsible for her husband's care 24/7, but a significant part of her life had ended, as did an identity that had been created by ten years of caregiving. In previous chapters, I wrote about the importance of understanding how your loved one's change in identity was affected by how important the loss was to her. Now it's your turn to examine how much you tied your identity to your loved one in the following four categories:

1. Work/professional role
2. Social relationships
3. Leisure activities
4. Intimacy

Work/professional role. Roles determine what we expect from others and what others expect from us. They embody the rules by which we live a significant part of our lives. A set of work expectations locks you in five or more days a week for at least nine hours a day. If your husband had little or nothing to do with your profession, this part of your life wouldn't be as affected as much as if he had been a business partner, as was the case with Anne, a woman who was married to the same man for fifteen years. They ran an email marketing company from their house. Decisions were always jointly made, and discussions about their business constantly occurred. With the death of her husband she felt as if a knife were cleaving her in two. She knew every aspect of the operation, so the emotion had nothing to do with her competence in running the business. Rather, she had lost a large part of her identity with the death of her husband.

Social Relationships

Some people believe that the most important variables for defining themselves are their relationships.[2] For many, they are the heart of their identity. It's irrelevant whether the relationships are good or terrible. What's critical is how dominating they are in their life. We are constantly interacting with others. If you are alive and not a hermit, you have social interactions. Many of them are mundane—such as the obligatory attendance at an office party—but others are important in defining who we are, as was the case for a devoted opera fan. Throughout his marriage, he and his wife attended every performance of the San Francisco Opera. When the season was over, they attended monthly social gatherings of friends, who like them, loved opera. An important part of his life vanished when his wife died. Overnight, the activity most important in his life was gone. He didn't miss going to the opera but rather going to the opera *with* his wife. He didn't miss the monthly social events to discuss opera but rather sitting *next to his wife* discussing *The Barber of Seville.*

Leisure Activities

You did many things by yourself before your loved one died, and other activities you did jointly. You may continue your solo enjoyable activities without experiencing a change in identity. But if you did the most enjoyable activities together, expect a change in the joy they will give you. Fellow kayakers suggested to a man who had spent almost every weekend with his wife traversing San Francisco Bay that he rejoin them for the weekly outings. They didn't understand that the activity he missed wasn't the two hours spent rowing from Sausalito to Angel Island but rather the time he had spent sliding through the water with the love of his life talking about their rich past and exciting future. Even tracing the exact water route couldn't bring back the emotion he had experienced with his wife.

Intimacy

Intimacy, whether physical or emotional, involves vulnerability. Your loved one shared with you parts of her life that were off limits to others, and you did the same with her. They could have been sexual behaviors that she may have been embarrassed to acknowledge with anyone other than you or emotions left unexplored with other people. A client and his wife had been best friends since their marriage forty years ago. Their intimacy had so much depth that when he started to say something, she would often finish the sentence and vice versa. After she died he would say something out loud and expect to have his sentence completed, but it never was.

Suggestions

1. There is no hierarchy for sorrow.
2. The more dependent a relationship with a lost loved one, the greater the grief.
3. The ending of a troubled relationship has the same effects on identity as the loss of a positive and loving one.

ACCEPTANCE AND MOVING FORWARD

The first step in moving on with your life is acceptance, but acceptance doesn't mean giving up or accepting the loss. Rather, acknowledge that the source of your lost emotion is gone but not your ability to experience the feeling he generated. The resurrection of joy can never happen by focusing on what you lost when your loved one died. The fixation with dwelling on loss baffled Thich Nhat Hanh. He couldn't understand why Western psychotherapists focused on what was wrong with people's lives rather than on what was exemplary.[3] I had witnessed the focus on the negative to solve problems in the 1970s when I lived south of Chicago.[4] People abandoned large swatches of the South Side when drug dealing, gang intimidation, and other activities began destroying the community. Community groups believed the problem could be solved by demolishing the abandoned buildings and fencing off areas where the buildings once stood. They assumed that once the negative influence was gone, something positive would soon replace it. Their efforts worked in reducing the violence but didn't lead to the construction of new homes. Positive change wouldn't occur for many years.

The lessons from Chicago's urban renewal apply to grief: spending time dwelling on your loss may not lead to the resurrection of lost emotions. I counseled a man who thought his soul mate had died because of medical incompetence. I asked when his wife had died. "Sixteen months, four days, and six hours ago," he said. "It was a Wednesday morning." He told me the only thing he wanted was "to make the pain stop." He had seen a psychiatrist for many months, supplemented by monthly attendance at a grief group and drugs to reduce his depression. In the individual and group sessions, the focus was on exploring the loss, not what could be done to resurrect his joy. It was the replication of my Chicago experience. The great seventeenth-century Japanese poet and samurai, Masahide, expressed an opposite approach to dealing with a loss. As a loyal servant of the emperor, he was ordered on a diplomatic journey. When he returned, he found that fire had destroyed his house. The tragedy became the basis for his most famous Haiku:

> Barn's burned down,
> Now I can see the moon.[5]

For Masahide, his loss represented an opportunity to experience something new. I know you can't envision the death of your loved one leading to the beginning of anything positive. You may feel guilty even contemplating anything positive coming from his death. Know that others, as was the case with Susan, exemplify a willingness to develop a new life. Her husband had died of leukemia, and she felt destined to remain alone forever. For months, she allowed the loss to reshape everything about her, from her interactions with fellow employees to those with her family and friends. She came to understand that the death of her husband wasn't the end of her life but rather the beginning of relationships and experiences that would have been impossible if he had lived. The playwright Tom Stoppard voiced the idea that losses aren't necessarily bad: "Every exit is an entrance somewhere else."[6] That's what acceptance is: the entry into a new life.

Suggestions

4. You'll need to accept your loss before you can move forward.
5. Shift your focus from the loss to what you wish to regain.

THERAPY: HOW MUCH TIME TO GRIEVE?

Everyone grieves differently, with solutions ranging from endless waiting to headlong rushes into new relationships. At the "waiting" end of the continuum are those who wait for the pain to subside on its own. An analogy is a person waiting at a remote train station. The stationmaster is gone, schedules aren't posted, and nobody is present to ask when he should expect the next train. So he waits. But for how long? A day? A week? A month? Many forms of grief therapy promote patience. Therapists maintain that the grief should dissipate naturally, but this waiting approach is unacceptable to many people who are experiencing grief. Imagine a dentist saying "Let's wait until the infected root in your tooth dissolves and then the pain will disappear." Or a pediatrician telling you that nothing needs to be done for your child who broke her arm because "in a month or two the

arm will heal and the pain will be gone." Neither your dentist nor pediatrician would give you this type of advice. Yet that's the premise of the *let's
wait for grief to dissipate* approach.

Another approach is to fill time with activities. In this approach, it's
hoped an abundance of things or actions over a period of time will reduce
the grief. You learned the futility of the approach in previous chapters
where I cautioned against filling your loved one's time with activities. My
mother's friends believed the best way of helping her overcome the grief
she experienced when my father died was to invite her to theater shows
and bring food to the house. They wanted my mother to pretend that life
went on and nothing had changed. They believed that with an endless
number of activities and the presence of friends, she would get over her
grief. They didn't understand that a road tour production of *My Fair Lady*
and coconut macaroons wouldn't replace someone she had lived with and
loved for forty years.

Somewhere along the continuum are counselors who believe in
Elizabeth Kübler-Ross's "step" theory on how to grieve a loss.[7] The
premise is that you will need to go through five stages of grieving before
you can put your loss behind you: denial, anger, bargaining, depression,
and acceptance. The journey may take years or sometimes a lifetime, as it
did for Lisa. Lisa's father had leukemia and died at a hospice facility where
I was a bedside volunteer. Two years after his death, Lisa's life remained
shattered. She attended regular sessions of a grief group that focused on
helping clients move through grief steps, and she saw a therapist for individual counseling every week. The focus in the group and individual
sessions was on the loss of her father. The group leader believed that the
pain would lessen if she traversed the five steps. Lisa wanted to focus on
her depression, but her therapist pulled her back to "anger" because he
believed that was the step on which she was stuck. Nobody explained to
Lisa how spending time thinking about and analyzing the loss and staying
in touch with the pain would result in the resurrection of the emotions
lost when her father died. Focusing on loss makes as much sense as a parent giving all her attention to one problem child while ignoring the needs
of her other children. I find waiting, filling time, and steps mystifying. In
the 1300s the Japanese poet Dōgen said a painting of a rice cake doesn't
help hunger.[8] I believe the same applies to grief. Both thinking and doing require energy. The more energy spent thinking, the less is available
for doing.

There is no "appropriate" amount of time regarding social mores or
effectiveness in getting over one's grief. So what makes the most sense

to you? Waiting until the grief leaves by itself? Moving the grief along through established steps? Finding something positive to replace the pain? Some counselors maintain that your choice of approaches should account for the long-term effects of grieving. In studies reported by Dr. Peter D. Cramer and others, clinical depression causes physical changes to the nerve pathways.[9] The longer depression lasts, the more likely physical damage will occur. In turn, the more the damage, the harder it becomes to get rid of depression. Depression is not common to all people who grieve, but distinctions between "clinical depression" and feeling lousy every day may be academic to those with disrupted lives.

What if you can't accept the train station analogy, the reasoning behind filling one's time, or the belief that overcoming grief requires a step approach? What if you wish to move through your loss as if you are on a speedboat rather than holding on to a half-submerged log? At the other end of the continuum are those who believe enduring the pain until it goes away makes no sense if other choices are available. People who adhere to this approach have adult children who often are baffled when a parent begins a new relationship after an "inappropriate" amount of time grieving. They believe grieving for an insufficient amount of time is disrespectful or an indication that there wasn't love between the person who died and the one who survived. Few people think their way out of grief. They need to *act*. We can't control certain events, including the circumstances of our loss. No matter what your lifestyle, nothing would have prevented your husband's lung cancer because he smoked before you met him. Once his cancer developed, you couldn't do anything as the cancer progressed, and his oncologist said he could do nothing further. We may not control events such as these, but we are in control of how the loss affects us. We can choose to allow the grief to persist and wait for the pain to subside, or we can do something to regain our joy. In John Lennon's song *Beautiful Boy*, he says life happens to you while you're busy making other plans.[10] I would change the lyrics to say life passes you by while you're busy grieving.

Suggestions

6. Don't expect rigid timelines for grief.
7. Don't use "steps" as an accurate way of determining where you are in the grief process.
8. Whatever approach to grief reduction you choose, account for the effect of time on the development of long-term depression.

LIVING IN THE PRESENT

Losses take you through all time zones: memories of what was, feelings you experience now, and visions of what will never happen. The resurrection of a lost emotion requires that you live in the present. If your grief is similar to that of many other people who have lost a loved one, you're spending an inordinate amount of time with memories and lamenting a nonexistent future, as was the case with a client who viewed every new relationship and experience as an inferior version of what he had experienced with his wife. His attempts to establish new relationships were doomed when he compared his present to his past life. No one could be as compassionate as his wife. No one could appreciate movies the way she did. No one could provide him with the care and love his wife did. When we focus on the past, idealized memories are created that leave out the negatives. This is one reason many awareness advocates maintain the importance of moving to the present: it avoids comparisons with idealized memories.[11] Moving into the present, however, is not sufficient for getting on with your life if everything about your awareness is negative. Focusing on the present should involve the search for skills, activities, and people with the potential for generating lost emotions, not replacing the person who died.

Suggestions

9. Shift your awareness from the past and future to the present.
10. Your awareness should focus on identifying skills, activities, and people having the potential to generate the emotions you no longer have.

IT TAKES ENERGY TO BE MISERABLE

People will often say they lack the energy necessary to do those activities that could give them joy. It takes the same amount of energy to be miserable as it does to be happy. Sometimes, even more effort is necessary to be miserable. Bill moped around the house for months, spending countless hours dwelling on the life he no longer had following the death of his partner. It was easier to watch reruns of sitcoms than to get on with his life. His lethargy was exhausting since it took effort to be miserable. "I'm too tired from my grief to do the things you're suggesting," Bill would say to me. He was right. He was so exhausted from dwelling on his losses that little energy remained for examining what was worthwhile in his life. I suggested that he could still spend time grieving but not as much. I tried to convince him to shift some of his energy to things he loved doing, like gardening.

"Why not spend ten minutes a day pulling weeds?" I suggested. "I understand how your grief incapacitates you, but can you stop doing it for ten minutes each day? If not, maybe ten minutes every other day?" He agreed to my request. He appeared different when I saw him the following week, smiling for the first time in months. "Whenever I went into the garden, I saw Jerry next to me pulling weeds and joking about my farming skills, and I wept. I wasn't sure if I could do it," he said. "You know, when I started pulling those weeds, I focused on them, not on my memories. It was wonderful. I'm now spending over an hour each day in the garden."

Two other things besides gardening were necessary before he could resurrect his joy. The first was taking a break from the hard work of mourning the loss of his partner. Second, he realized other things in life could bring back the peacefulness he had experienced before Jerry's death. Over 2,000 years ago, the Buddha supposedly said that you are today because of what you did in the past but that your future is dependent only on what you do now.[12] The message, which is as relevant today as it was when he first said it, is that the past becomes the future only if you do nothing to change it in the present. View the past as a painting drawn on water, and you will begin taking control of your life. Bill's simple act of pulling weeds began the healing. If you do nothing to reenter the present, you will, in the words of Pema Chodron, be riding backward on a train—seeing where you have been but not where you are going.[13]

Suggestion

11. Take frequent breaks from your grief by focusing on something simple and concrete.

FINDING THE LOST EMOTION

You may believe that nothing can take the place of your loved one. For many losses, the inability to find a substitute is more apparent than real. Of course, you can't replace a loved one who shared your life for fifty years, but *you can replace the emotion she created in you.* You won't find it easy to identify the emotion since we don't think in specific terms of why we miss someone. The usual response to grief is "I just miss him," or "We were inseparable," or "She was my best friend." One client needed time to determine what it was about her husband that had made her joyful. We examined some areas, but nothing appeared right until she realized what had made him endearing was how he had encouraged her potential for creativity. She stopped trying to replace him and explored activities that could replicate what she had felt when they took craft lessons together. Spending a week at a school of folk arts put her on the path of recreating the joy she had experienced with her husband. You need first to determine, as my client did, the emotion you wish to recover, and then explore activities for its regeneration.

Regaining one lost emotion doesn't automatically lead to recovering another. For example, my client recovered the joy of being creative but knew there were other emotions that required separate activities, such as intimacy. If your losses are multiple, as they were for my client, focus on one emotion, since the activities you will be choosing for each may be different. My suggestion is to choose the emotion you are grieving the least since it will pose fewer recovery problems. For example, the death of a client's husband led to the loss of physical intimacy, social companionship, humor, and sharing. Of the four emotions, my client believed that sharing would be the easiest to resurrect and intimacy the most difficult. He started on "sharing" by joining a group of people who were mourning the loss of a partner and worked his way down the list. The emotion you choose shouldn't be too general (e.g., happiness). To paraphrase Alfred North Whitehead, we aspire in generalities but live in a world of specifics. I want to be "happy," but achieving happiness requires the completion of specific activities. For me, it's getting six hours of sleep a night, writing for five hours a day, playing my flute every day, taking my dog for a walk on the beach, and having meaningful conversations with my wife. Those are the specifics of my happiness. I can't *be* happy, but I can *do* things that *enable* me to be happy.

The journey to happiness is different for everyone. You may have tried a path in the past and failed. With each failure, you thought it was your fault. Most likely, it wasn't. *Your failures in recovering joy are related more to a lack of knowledge than to anything in your personality or level of motivation.* There was nothing wrong with you. Rather, you didn't possess the information necessary to be successful. You knew *what* you wanted to resurrect but not *how* to do it. Knowing what you wish to change without knowing how to do it is like attempting to cross a swift river in a rowboat without oars.

Suggestions

12. Choose one emotion for recovery that poses the least difficulties.
13. Don't confine your search to people. Skills and activities can also generate the lost emotion.

14. Don't assume that regaining one feeling will lead to recovering other emotions.
15. Be specific regarding the emotions you want to recover.

UNIVERSAL PRINCIPLES FOR RESURRECTING JOY

For many years, I and other researchers in the social and clinical sciences have documented how the use of certain universal principles result in change, regardless of the characteristics of the person wishing to change or the type of change sought.[14] Some of these involve simple ideas, such as focusing on only one goal at a time. Others are more complex, like making new attitudes automatic. I began applying these strategies more than twenty-five years ago in clinical situations. The results were surprising to my clients and me. They were able to do behaviors unimaginable only months before therapy or coaching began. Some examples are a woman traumatized by an accident again took pleasure in driving. A child whose language was delayed learned new linguistic structures. A woman who had a stroke and had difficulty retrieving words learned a memory strategy allowing her to communicate. The principles are:

1. All behaviors are complex.
2. Change is frightening.
3. Change must be positive.
4. Being is easier than becoming.
5. Slower is better.
6. Know more, do better.
7. Change requires structure.
8. Practice is necessary.
9. Protect new behaviors.
10. Small changes are big.

Think of the principles as ten feeder streams leading into a river. As each flows, the river's current increases. Just as the river's current is dependent on the number of sources and their incoming flow, so will the magnitude of your successes be dependent on the number of principles you choose to use. I found the resurrection of emotions related to the number of principles my clients used.[15] The more principles you use, the greater will be your successes.

All Behaviors are Complex

When we think of the emotion we want to recover, our thoughts tend to be global. For example, you don't miss *traveling* with your husband but rather a sense of *fulfillment* that was present when you were with him. For a client who had lost his wife, the re-creation of "stability" was important. But what are the components of stability? For him it involved creating an exercise schedule he would adhere to, organizing his house, designating certain days to do specific chores, and visiting museums weekly. The combination of all these activities constituted the components of stability. He didn't search for "stability" but rather focused on the completion of four activities that would lead to stability.

Change is Frightening

Change is frightening, whether it's coming to terms with being a widow or looking at a confusing pile of bills. You were forced to give up a world you knew for an unknown one. The death of your loved one dragged you, kicking and screaming, from a life as comfortable as an old easy chair into a strange new world. Your life became analogous to a large boulder balanced on a precipice. It looks like it could tumble off the cliff if a little pressure were applied. Despite your considerable effort, it won't budge. The weight and inertia of the boulder prevent it from moving. And as with the boulder, inertia prevents us from accepting our new world. We are all resistant to change, even when we say we are not. You may be moving from dependence to independence, being in control to having little of it, and giving up significant parts of your life for a void. Nobody asks you whether it's acceptable to move from A to B. There is discomfort in most transitions, sometimes even fear, especially when the movement is taking you from a familiar identity to one still forming. You can make change less frightening by doing some simple things. Whatever goals you wish to achieve, make them more realistic, smaller, and sequential. Each subsequent step in the recovery process should be slightly harder than what preceded it. By doing these things, the fear of change can be reduced.

Change Must be Positive

We rarely develop new behaviors or attitudes if they aren't more positive than negative. Three types of rewards for change can be present: the act of doing an activity, its completion, and a payoff.[16] The *act of doing* something can be rewarding enough to make change happen, regardless of how rewarding the outcome or how big the payoff. An example is the client I referred to earlier who found pulling weeds enjoyable as a break from grieving. The second type of reward involves the *completion of an act*. My client was delighted with the look of the garden when he had finished weeding. The third type of reward is the *payoff*, which is something not directly related to the act or its completion. In our gardening example, it would be people passing by and commenting on how good the yard looks. The best combination for changing behaviors leading to the resurrection of emotions is a combination of the three.

Being is Easier Than Becoming

The law of inertia applies to the movement of physical objects as well as to the difficulty of changing emotions. The businessperson and philanthropist W. Clement Stone warned, "So many fail because they don't get started—they don't go. They don't overcome inertia. They don't begin."[17] Objects at rest want to stay at rest. Familiar emotions want to continue regardless of whether they are positive or painful.

There's a story of a moaning dog lying on the front porch of a house. Next to the dog sits an old man in a rocking chair, whittling a piece of wood. A stranger comes by and is confused by the scene. He walks up to the porch to see what the problem is with the dog.

"Howdy, neighbor," he says to the old man.

"Howdy," the old man responds, not looking up from the piece of wood he's carving.

"I was wondering why your hound is yelping."

"He's lying on a nail," the old man says, taking a puff on his corncob pipe.

"How long's he been doing that?" the stranger asks.

"Oh, I reckon about eight hours."

"Eight hours!" the shocked stranger says.

"Yup."

"Well, why doesn't he get off it?"

The old man stops whittling, takes another puff on his pipe, and strokes his beard as if in deep thought. He looks up at the stranger and says, "I guess he forgot what it's like not lying on it."

Just like the old hound dog, we fear change's double-edged sword: giving up the known while accepting the unknown. Two strategies are suggested to overcome the inertia. The first is that when given options, choose an easier path. The motto "no pain, no gain" may be appropriate for those believing in a macho credo of life, but it's a failure formula for the resurrection of a lost emotion. Too much pain, and the status quo wins out. Like the hound dog, your fear of what might replace the pain may keep it a constant companion. A client identified the lost emotion he wished to regain as "a sense of peacefulness." He embraced the "no pain, no gain" motto and decided to spend an entire day at an isolated place in a park where he and his wife had spent many enjoyable afternoons. Everything was fine for the first fifteen minutes. Most of the memories were pleasant, and even those that weren't, were tolerable. Despite being anxious, he decided to remain, assuming nothing would change, but it did. With each minute, the painful memories of her loss outpaced the pleasant ones. After three hours he fled the park, more depressed than he had been in months. The lesson is that change should be easy and gentle. He would have left the park with a sense of peacefulness if he had stayed for only ten minutes. Ending an activity with positive thoughts is an essential step for recovering an emotion.

The second strategy is to avoid boredom. Boredom develops when something is repetitive or done for too long. Even if you are successful, the new behavior doesn't last. An example is a client who chose to volunteer at a local hospital as a way of regaining a sense of purpose. The only position open was as an assistant to the manager of the gift shop. She moved stock instead of doing anything meaningful. After volunteering two days a week for three weeks, she left. The activity couldn't provide meaningful interactions for her, and if it could, boredom could still develop based on the length of time she was there and the number of days.

Slower is Better

We value quickness as a society and lack the patience for allowing things to develop slowly and systematically. This shortsighted expectation applies to our bodies, careers, financial status, and a host of other things including resurrecting lost emotions. Research shows that the quick acquisition of new behaviors is less stable than one developed over a longer period.[18] One strategy that moves actions along is called *successive approximations*.[19] The procedure involves the systematic and slow journeying to a distant goal. Unlike Kübler-Ross's grieving steps, there is ample research evidence that it works.[20] Take the example of the person who fled the park more anxious when he left than when he had entered. He should have started with ten minutes the first day and increased the length by five minutes during each visit. Incremental changes can also involve gradual increases in effort, the number of component behaviors, and skill level. The path of change should be slow, with each step leading you closer to the resurrection of the lost emotion.

Know More, Do Better

Mysteries and surprises are necessary ingredients for novels but disastrous for recovering emotions. You can reduce the uncertainty of change and increase the probability of success if you know how change occurs. Two effective strategies are monitoring and explanatory feedback. Monitoring is an ongoing process that informs a person about how well the change is progressing. It involves anything that indicates movement toward a goal. An example is a woman who became negative with friends after her husband's death. She wanted to be as positive a person as she was before he died, but she couldn't tell when her "tone" became negative. After discussing the problem with a friend, they decided that whenever she became negative, her friend would twirl her necklace. By monitoring her behavior, she was able to increase the number of positive interactions.

Explanatory feedback goes beyond monitoring. It provides an analysis of an activity. After the death of his wife, a middle management executive was having problems supervising his employees. He wanted to regain the joy he had experienced at work before his wife died but couldn't understand why it wasn't redeveloping. For a short period, he asked his supervisor, who was a friend, to observe his interactions and provide him with feedback on how he was supervising his employees. They agreed that feedback would focus on three areas: tone, conversational flow, and labeling statements that were positive or negative. With explanatory feedback, an analysis involves correcting problems rather than affixing blame for failures. Knowledge about the path facilitates the resurrection of the lost emotion.

Change Requires Structure

Many people view structure as restrictive, something that inhibits spontaneity. Spontaneity is wonderful for some activities but a surefire method for sabotaging the resurrection of an emotion. Lost emotions rarely spontaneously develop, and if they do, their duration is short. Practice schedules shouldn't be rigid but rather modifiable if they no longer work. Events should be sequenced since sometimes the key to success involves the order in which the steps are performed.[21] For example, following her son's death, a woman who lectured worldwide had difficulty speaking at conferences. She began reengaging by publically speaking during the morning for one month since this was the time when she was least affected by her grief. After the successful completion of the activity, she began lecturing in the afternoons and then in the evenings, the time when her grief was most intense. Structure doesn't limit spontaneity; rather, it provides a platform for the resurrection of emotions, which, once established, can become spontaneous.

Practice is Necessary

The idea of practicing an emotion may sound ludicrous, but according to the great dancer and choreographer Martha Graham, it's no different than practicing a motor or cognitive skill. She said, "We learn by practice. Whether it means to learn to dance by practicing dancing or to learn to live by practicing living."[22] People often associate the term "practice" with a boring and repetitive activity. Yet practice is the basis of change in almost every activity.[23] Few people think of practice as a necessary component for the resurrection of an emotion, but it is. Strategies can involve increasing the amount of time spent doing something, varying the time and days, and selecting who or what generates the emotion. A woman had difficulty initiating conversations after her partner died. She decided to practice warm greetings by starting with salespeople, and then she moved on to practicing with her friends when the behavior had become automatic with strangers. By integrating the emotion into everyday life, the ability to initiate conversations became automatic. Practice sessions mimicking reality can produce automaticity. For example, use a simplified version of the emotion you wish to develop (e.g., enjoyment instead of love). Practice is not something isolated from our everyday life. Integrating the emotion into normal activities is more likely to result in permanent behavioral and emotional changes.

Protect New Behaviors

Associations trigger emotions. An example is someone who is grieving the death of her husband. She reverts to despondency whenever she visits a nearby city where he had proposed to her. Even though she had attempted to develop new relationships, visiting the area ended them. Associations with the status quo emotion may be so strong that they prevent the resurrection of the lost one. Methods for identifying associations include doing an inventory of objects, events, and people associated with the status quo emotion, followed by methods of desensitization (the stimulus no longer evokes a painful reaction).[24]

Resurrected emotions need new associations to survive.[25] They'll wither and disappear if you learn them in isolation since a recovered emotion's associations are few and weak. You'll need to strengthen associations if the emotion is to persist. Strategies include the use of rewards and the conscious pairing of the new emotion with objects, events, and people. Think of your new emotions as if they were as fragile as a baby bird.

Small Changes Are Big

There is an old saying that failure spreads like rust on an unattended boat. The bigger the goal, the lower the probability of success. Little successes, however, are like amorous bunnies—the more of them you have, the more of them you'll get. To paraphrase a popular line, success is the gift that keeps on giving. Strive for the completion of small goals rather than reaching for the "brass ring." For example, an objective for a man grieving the loss of social interaction is mingling at a party—an unreachable goal unless he starts with small chunks of time. He began attending a social event close to when it was scheduled to end. Mingling for ten minutes was easy compared to interacting with people for the full two hours. After completing the small goal, the next goal was fifteen minutes, then twenty, and so on until he felt comfortable for the entire duration of an event. Little successes, such as these, often lead to the "big one" with little or no effort. Everyone wants to do things in a "big" way: big jobs, big money, and big successes. Attempts at achieving big successes often result in big failures, which deplete one's reservoir of self-esteem. Little successes, which are easier to complete, replenish the pool. Forget about achieving "big things." They will materialize by themselves if you do the steps leading to them with awareness and appreciation.

Suggestions

16. Don't keep reaching for the "brass ring." You'll fail more than you'll succeed.
17. The completion of each small goal becomes the stepping-stone to your next objective.
18. Assume that the emotion you are trying to resurrect is complex.
19. Since change is frightening, do whatever is necessary to reduce the discomfort, including selecting smaller and more realistic goals.
20. Whatever you want to change should result in a positive outcome. If it does not, the new behavior or attitude will disappear.
21. Change should be almost as easy as not changing.
22. For change to be long lasting, it should be developed slowly.
23. The more you know about the principles of change, the more likely you will be successful.

24. Your attempts to recover an emotion should be structured.
25. If the new emotion is to become stable, it requires practice.
26. Develop associations for the resurrected emotions.
27. Striving for many small successes is better than continually failing by looking for only "big" successes.

TROUBLESHOOTING

Many people focus on assessing blame when failures happen. This backward-looking approach to life interferes with the re-creation of joy. Don't blame yourself. Rather, view every failure as an opportunity to learn how to do something differently. The less time spent blaming yourself and others, the more time is available for determining what should change the next time you attempt the activity. The process of change is ongoing, with the resurrection of an emotion taking months or years. Instead of looking at final goals, ask the questions "Am I closer to my goal today than I was last week? Am I enjoying the journey?" Even though you didn't accomplish everything you set out to change, life continues to evolve—as does the resurrection of emotions. The "new you" is someone in transition. You will always be evolving.

Suggestions

28. Don't blame yourself for failures. Failures are opportunities to learn.
29. You will always be in transition.

NOTES

CHAPTER 1

1. "Cancer Statistics," *National Cancer Institute* (2015), http://www.cancer.gov/about-cancer/what-is-cancer/statistics.

2. M. Merleau-Ponty, *Phenomenology of Perception*, trans. Colin Smith (London: Routledge, 1962).

3. Thelonious Monk, *Monk's Dream*, Sony Records, 2002.

4. Stephen Thomas Erlewine, *Song Review by Stephen Thomas Erlewine*, http://www.allmusic.com/song/bright-mississippi-mt0003455227.

5. Peter Lattman, "The Origins of Justice Stewart's 'I Know It When I See It,'" *LawBlog at The Wall Street Journal Online* (September 27, 2007), http://blogs.wsj.com/law/2007/09/27/the-origins-of-justice-stewarts-i-know-it-when-i-see-it/.

6. Thich Nhat Hanh, *No Death, No Fear* (New York: Riverhead, 2002).

7. The Dali Lama, *An Open Heart: Practicing Compassion in Everyday Life* (New York: Back Bay Books, 2002).

8. Stan Goldberg, "How Can I Be a Compassionate Caregiver?" *Buddhadharma*, Winter (2011): 64–69.

9. Leigh Montville, *Evel: The High-Flying Life of Evel Knievel: American Showman, Daredevil, and Legend* (New York: Anchor, 2012).

10. Martin Hackworth, "The Physics of Motorcycles," *Motorcyclejazz.com*, http://www.motorcyclejazz.com/motorcycle_physics.htm.

11. Jacob Bronowski, *The Ascent of Man* (Boston: Brown, 1974).

12. William Shakespeare, *The Merchant of Venice* (New York: Simon & Schuster, 2009), Act 4, scene 1, p. 190.

13. Stanley A. Goldberg, *Clinical Skills for Speech-Language Pathologists: Practical Applications* (San Diego: Singular, 1996).

14. *Rashomon*, DVD, directed by Akira Kurosawa (1950; Tokyo: The Criterion Collection).

15. Daniel L. Schacter, ed., *How Minds, Brains, and Societies Reconstruct the Past* (Boston: Harvard University Press, 1997).

16. Lewis White Beck, ed., *Eighteenth-Century Philosophy: Readings in the History of Philosophy* (New York: Free Press, 1966).

17. Stan Goldberg, *Lessons for the Living: Stories of Forgiveness, Gratitude, and Courage at the End of Life* (Boston: Trumpeter, 2013).

18. "Cancer Statistics," *National Cancer Institute*, 2015, http://www.cancer.gov/about-cancer/what-is-cancer/statistics.

19. Stan Goldberg, "Welcome to Kauai: What's That Strange Stick in Your Hand?" *Saltwater Fly Fishing*, December (1999): 22–27.

20. John Lennon, *Walls and Bridges*, © 2010 by EMI, compact disc.

21. Alfred Korzybski, *Science and Sanity: An Introduction to Non-Aristotelian Systems and General Semantics*, 5th ed. (New York: Institute of General Semantics, 1995).

22. Sogyal Rinpoche, *Tibetan Wisdom for Living and Dying* (Louisville, CO: Sounds True, 2006). Audiotape.

23. "Prostate Cancer," *NIH Research*, http://report.nih.gov/nihfactsheets/ViewFactSheet.aspx?csid=60.

24. Groucho Marx, *Groucho and Me* (Boston: Da Capo Press, 1959), 321.

25. "Cancer Statistics," *National Cancer Institute*, 2015, http://www.cancer.gov/about-cancer/what-is-cancer/statistics.

26. A. W. Partin et al., "Combination of Prostate-Specific Antigen, Clinical Stage, and Gleason Score to Predict Pathological Stage of Localized Prostate Cancer: A Multi-Institutional Update," *JAMA* 277, no. 18 (1997): 1445–1451.

27. Howard M. Sandler et al., "Overall Survival After Prostate-Specific-Antigen-Detected Recurrence Following Conformal Radiation Therapy," *International Journal of Radiation Oncology* 48, no. 3 (2000): 629–633.

28. J. R. Stark et al., "Gleason Score and Lethal Prostate Cancer: Does 3 + 4 = 4 + 3?" *Journal of Clinical Oncology* 27, no. 21 (2009): 3459–3464.

29. Y. Chavan, *Meditation for Beginners: How to Relieve Stress, Anxiety and Depression and Return to a State of Inner Peace and Happiness*, CreateSpace, 2014.

30. F. Zeldan et al., "Neural Correlates of Mindfulness Meditation-Related Anxiety Relief," *Social Cognitive and Affective Neuroscience* 9, no. 6 (2013) doi: 10.1093/scan/nst041.

31. Goldberg, *Clinical Skills for Speech-Language Pathologists*.

CHAPTER 2

1. Stan Goldberg, "Now the Bad News," *Shambhala Sun Magazine*, July (2013): 47–48.

2. Adam Alter, "Why It's Dangerous to Label People," *Psychology Today*, May 17 (2010), https://www.psychologytoday.com/blog/alternative-truths/201005/why-its-dangerous-label-people.

3. John B. Carroll, ed., *Language, Thought, and Reality: Selected Writings of Benjamin Lee Whorf* (Boston: MIT Press, 1964).

4. Stan Goldberg, "When You Can't Let Go," *Shambhala Sun Magazine*, May (2012): 47–49.

5. S. Uttam et al., "Early Prediction of Cancer Progression by Depth-Resolved Nanoscale Maps of Nuclear Architecture from Unstained Tissue Specimens," *Cancer Research* 75, no. 22 (2015): 4718–4727.

6. Carlos Castaneda, *The Teachings of Don Juan: A Yaqui Way of Knowledge.* (New York: Washington Square Press, 1985).

7. S. Milazzo, S. Lejeune, and E. Ernst, "Laetrile for Cancer: A Systematic Review of the Clinical Evidence," *Supportive Care in Cancer* 15, no. 6 (2007): 532–505. doi: 10.1007/s00520-006-0168-9.

8. Carl Sagan and Ann Druyan, *The Demon-Haunted World: Science as a Candle in the Dark* (New York: Ballantine Books, 1997).

9. J. Simons, "Prostate Cancer Immunotherapy: Beyond Immunity to Curability," *Cancer Immunology Research* 2, no. 11 (2014): 1034.

10. A. Molassiotis et al., "Use of Complementary and Alternative Medicine in Cancer Patients: A European Survey, *Annals of Oncology* 16, no. 4 (2005): 655–663.

11. "W. C. Fields Biography." *IMDb.* http://www.imdb.com/name/nm000 1211/bio.

12. "Types of Cancer Treatments and Care," *U.S. Food and Drug Administration.* Last updated 6/19/15. http://www.fda.gov/forpatients/illness/cancer/ucm 408053.htm. http://www.fda.gov/forpatients/illness/cancer/ucm408053.htm

13. Walter Isaacson, *Steve Jobs* (New York: Simon & Schuster, 2015).

14. Andrew Weil, "Did Steve Jobs Get Good Cancer Treatment?" *DrWeil. com,* http://www.drweil.com/drw/u/QAA401029/Did-Steve-Jobs-Get-Good -Cancer-Treatment.html.

15. Christopher K. Daugherty and Fay J. Hlubocky, "What Are Terminally Ill Cancer Patients Told About Their Expected Deaths? A Study of Cancer Physicians' Self-Reports of Prognosis Disclosure," *Journal of Clinical Oncology* 26, no. 36 (2008): 5988–5993. doi: 10.1200/JCO.2008.17.2221.

16. Karen Hancock et al., "Truth-Telling in Discussing Prognosis in Advanced Life-Limiting Illnesses: A Systematic Review," *Palliative Medicine* 21 (2007): 507–517.

17. Neelam Saleem Punjani, "Truth Telling to Terminally Ill Patients: To Tell or Not to Tell," *Journal of Clinical Research & Bioethics* 4 (2015): 159. doi: 10.4172/2155-9627.1000159.

18. P. Ginestier, *Anouilh* (Paris: Seghers, 1974).

19. Stan Goldberg, "What Makes You Think You'll Live Forever?" *Buddhadharma,* Fall (2010): 69–71.

20. Stefan Welz, Maximilian Nyazi, Claus Belka, and Ute Ganswindt, "Surgery vs. Radiotherapy in Localized Prostate Cancer: Which Is Best?" *Radiation Oncology* 3, no. 23 (2008): 23.

21. John E. Sarno, *The Mindbody Prescription: Healing the Body, Healing the Pain* (New York: Warner Books, 1999).

22. "Cancer Treatment & Survivorship Facts & Figures," *American Cancer Society,* 2015, http://www.cancer.org/research/cancerfactsstatistics/survivor-facts-figures.

23. N. Howlander et al., eds., "SEER Cancer Statistics Review, 1975-2012," *National Cancer Institute*. Last updated 11/18/15. http://seer.cancer.gov/csr/1975_2012/.

24. D. Cline et al., *Tintinalli's Emergency Medicine Manual,* 7th ed. (New York: McGraw-Hill Education, 2012).

25. "Depression," *National Cancer Institute*, http://www.cancer.gov/about-cancer/coping/feelings/depression-pdq-section/all.

26. C. McGrath et al., "Toward a Neuroimaging Treatment Selection Biomarker for Major Depressive Disorder," *JAMA Psychiatry* 70, no. 8 (2013): 821–829. doi: 10.1001/jamapsychiatry.2013.143.

27. Joanne Reeve, Mari Lloyd-Williams, and Chris Dowrick, "Depression in Terminal Illness: The Need for Primary Care-Specific Research," *Family Practice* 24, no. 3 (2007): 263–268. doi: 10.1093/fampra/cmm017.

28. A. Centena and G. Onik, *Prostate Cancer: A Patient's Guide to Treatment* (Omaha, NE: Addicus Books, 2014).

29. R. Foote et al., "The Clinical Case for Proton Beam Therapy," *Radiation Oncology* 7 (2012): 174. doi: 10.1186/1748-717X-7-174.

30. Thomas A. D'Amico, "Outcomes After Surgery for Esophageal Cancer," *Gastrointestinal Cancer Research* 1, no. 5 (2007): 188–196.

31. "Statistics and Outlook for Oesophageal Cancer," *Cancer Research UK*, http://www.cancerresearchuk.org/about-cancer/type/oesophageal-cancer/treatment/statistics-and-outlook-for-oesophageal-cancer.

32. P. Rochigneux et al., "Radio(Chemo)Therapy in Elderly Patients with Esophageal Cancer: A Feasible Treatment with an Outcome Consistent with Younger Patients," *Frontiers in Oncology*, 4 (2014). http://dx.doi.org/10.3389/fonc.2014.00100.

33. Alexander D. Karatzanis et al., "Management of Locally Advanced Laryngeal Cancer," *Journal of Otolaryngology-Head & Neck Surgery* 43 (2014): 4. doi: 10.1186/1916-0216-43-4.

34. Siew Tzuh Tang and Shiu-Yu C. Lee, "Cancer Diagnosis and Prognosis in Taiwan: Patient Preferences Versus Experiences," *Psycho-Oncology* 13, no. 1 (2004): 1–13.

CHAPTER 3

1. Zhiyuan Shen, "Genomic Instability and Cancer: An Introduction," *Journal of Molecular Cell Biology* 3, no. 1 (2011) 1–3.

2. "Types of Treatment," *National Cancer Institute*, http://www.cancer.gov/about-cancer/treatment/types.

3. Maarten Hofman et al., "Cancer-Related Fatigue: The Scale of the Problem," *The Oncologist* 12 Supplement 1 (2007): 4–10.

4. Anthony J. Bazzon et al., "Diet and Nutrition in Cancer Survivorship and Palliative Care," *Evidence-Based Complementary and Alternative Medicine Volume 2013*, http://dx.doi.org/10.1155/2013/917647.

5. Maarten Hofman et al., "Cancer-Related Fatigue: The Scale of the Problem."

6. Nancy E. Adler and Ann E. K. Page, eds., *Cancer Care for the Whole Patient: Meeting Psychosocial Health Needs* (Washington, DC: National Academies Press, 2008).

7. F. Cardoso et al., "Locally Recurrent or Metastatic Breast Cancer: ESMO Clinical Practice Guidelines for Diagnosis, Treatment and Follow-Up," *Annuals of Oncology* 23, no. 7 (2012): 11–19 doi: 10.1093/annonc/mds232.

8. John P. Cunha, ed., "Femara Side Effects Center," *RxList: The Internet Drug Index*. Last updated 5/22/15. http://www.rxlist.com/femara-side-effects-drug-center.htm.

9. Kevin T. Nead et al., "Androgen Deprivation Therapy and Future Alzheimer's Disease Risk," *Journal of Clinical Oncology* 34, no. 6 (2016): 566–571. doi: 10.1200/JCO.2015.63.6266.

10. W. M. van der Filler and P. Scheltens, "Epidemiology and Risk Factors of Dementia," *Journal of Neurology, Neurosurgery & Psychiatry* 76, no. 5 (2005): 2–7. doi:10.1136/jnnp.2005.082867.

11. G. Davey Smith and S. Ebrahim, eds., "Hormone Replacement Therapy (HRT): Risks and Benefits," *International Journal of Epidemiology* 30, no. 3 (2001): 423–426. doi: 10.1093/ije/30.3.423.

12. Neil Greenberg, James A. Carr, and Cliff H. Summers, "Causes and Consequences of Stress," *Integrative & Comparative Biology* 42, no. 3 (2002): 508–516. doi: 10.1093/icb/42.3.508.

13. David Schiller, *The Little Zen Companion* (New York: Workman Publishing, 1994): 133.

14. Jane Turner and Brian Kelly, "Emotional Dimensions of Chronic Disease," *Western Journal of Medicine* 172, no. 2 (2000): 124–128.

15. Liza Varvogli and Christina Darviri, "Stress Management Techniques: Evidence-Based Procedures That Reduce Stress and Promote Health," *Health Science Journal* 5, no. 2 (2011): 74–89.

16. Nancy E. Adler and Ann E. K. Page, eds., *Cancer Care for the Whole Patient: Meeting Psychosocial Health Needs* (Washington, DC: National Academies Press, 2008).

17. Stan Goldberg, "The Hard Work of Dying," *Shambhala Sun* November (2009): 27–29.

18. Stan Goldberg, "When You Can't Let Go," *stangoldbergwriter.com*, http://stangoldbergwriter.com/about/when-you-cant-let-go/.

19. Sogyal Rinpoche, *The Tibetan Book of Living and Dying* (London: Rider & Company, 1996).

20. Stan Goldberg, *Leaning into Sharp Points: Practical Guidance and Nurturing Support for Caregivers* (Novato, CA: New World Library, 2012).

21. "Side Effects of Hormone Therapy," *Prostate Cancer Foundation*, http://www.pcf.org/site/c.leJRIROrEpH/b.5836631/k.3CD9/Side_Effects_of_Hormone_Therapy.htm.

22. Thomas J. Meyer and Melvin M. Mark, "Effects of Psychosocial Interventions with Adult Cancer Patients: A Meta-Analysis of Randomized Experiments," *Health Psychology* 14, no. 2 (1995): 101–108. http://dx.doi.org/10.1037/0278-6133.14.2.101.

23. Karen Lawson and Sue Towey, "What Lifestyle Changes Are Recommended for Anxiety and Depression?" *University of Minnesota Center for Spirituality & Healing*, http://www.takingcharge.csh.umn.edu/manage-health-conditions/anxiety-depression/what-lifestyle-changes-are-recommended-anxiety-and-depre.

CHAPTER 4

1. Mark R. Leary and June Price Tangney, *Handbook of Self and Identity* (New York: Guilford Press, 2003).

2. David D. Burns, *The Feeling Good Handbook* (New York: Plume, 1999).

3. Stan Goldberg, "How Can I Be a Compassionate Caregiver?" *Buddhadharma* Winter (2001): 64–68.

4. Rick DelVecchio, "Witness to Death's Spirituality," *Catholic San Francisco*, July 8, 2009, http://www.catholic-sf.org/news_select.php?newsid=23&id=56182.

5. Stan Goldberg, "Learning From Our Losses," *Living with Loss Magazine* 24, no. 4 (2009): 36–37.

6. Stan Goldberg, "The 10 Rules of Change, *Psychology Today*. Last updated 12/4/12. https://www.psychologytoday.com/articles/200210/the-10-rules-change.

7. Stan Goldberg, *Lessons for the Living: Stories of Forgiveness, Gratitude, and Courage at the End of Life* (Boston: Trumpeter, 2009).

8. "World Cancer Day 2013—Global Press Release," *worldcancerday.org,* http://www.worldcancerday.org/world-cancer-day-2013-global-press-release.

9. Ibid.

10. Nancy E. Adler and Ann E. K. Page, eds., *Cancer Care for the Whole Patient: Meeting Psychosocial Health Needs* (Washington, DC: National Academies Press, 2008).

11. Sarah Knapp, Allison Marziliano, and Anne Moyer, "Identity Threat and Stigma in Cancer Patients," *Health Psychology Open* 1, no. 1 (2014): doi: 10.1177/2055102914552281.

12. Dhruba Deb, "Understanding the Unpredictability of Cancer Using Chaos Theory and Modern Art Techniques," *Leonardo* 49, no. 1 (2016): 66–67. doi: 10.1162/LEON_a_01099.

CHAPTER 5

1. Stan Goldberg, "Understanding Patients' Behaviors," *Hospice Volunteer News*, 3rd quarter (2009).

2. Sogyal Rinpoche, *Living Well, Dying Well* (Louisville, CO: Sounds True, 1993). Audiobook.

3. Michal Ephratt, "The Functions of Silence, *Journal of Pragmatics* 40 (2008): 1909–1938, http://www.gloriacappelli.it/wp-content/uploads/2009/05/silence.pdf.

4. Anthony L. Back, Susan M. Bauer-Wu, Cynda H. Rushton, and Joan Halifax, "Compassionate Silence in the Patient-Clinician Encounter: A Contemplative Approach," *Journal of Palliative Medicine* 12, no. 12 (2009): 1113–1117. doi: 10.1089/jpm.2009.0175.

5. "San Bruno Gas Explosion News," *ABCNews*, http://abcnews.go.com/topics/news/san-bruno-gas-explosion.htm.

6. Stan Goldberg, *Ready to Learn: How to Help Your Preschooler Succeed* (New York: Oxford University Press, 2005).

7. S. Goldberg, "Being Present at the Bedside," in *Communication and Positive Counseling*, ed. A. Holland (San Diego: Plural Publications, 2007).

8. Tulio Maranhao, *The Interpretation of Dialogue* (Chicago: University of Chicago Press, 1990).

9. Namkje Koudenburg, Tom Postmes, and Ernestine H. Gordijn, "Conversational Flow Promotes Solidarity," *PLoS One* 8, no. 11 (2013): e78363. doi: 10.1371/journal.pone.0078363.

10. Goldberg, *Ready to Learn*.

11. Stanley A. Goldberg, *Clinical Skills for Speech-Language Pathologists: Practical Applications* (San Diego: Singular, 1997).

12. Koudenburg et al., "Conversational Flow Promotes Solidarity."

13. Deborah Cameron, *Working with Spoken Discourse* (London: SAGE, 2001).

14. Goldberg, *Clinical Skills for Speech-Language Pathologists*.

15. Jacques Mehler, Josiane Bertoncini, and Michele Barriere, "Infant Recognition of Mother's Voice," *Perception*, 7 (1978): 491–497, https://www.sissa.it/cns/Articles/78infantRecognitionOfMothersVoice.pdf.

16. Jesse Snedeker and John Trueswell, "Using Prosody to Avoid Ambiguity: Effects of Speaker Awareness and Referential Context," *Journal of Memory and Language* [Internet]. 48 (2003): 103–130.

17. Mark G. Frank, Andreas Maroulis, and Darrin J. Griffin, "The Voice," in *Nonverbal Communication: Science and Applications*, ed. David Matsumoto, Mark Frank, and Hyi Sung Hwan (Washington, DC: SAGE, 2013), 53–74.

18. Graham McGregor, "Intonation and Meaning in Conversation," *Language & Communication* 2, no. 2 (1982): 123–131.

19. Bella M. DePaulo, "Nonverbal Behavior and Self-Presentation," *Psychological Bulletin* 111, no. 2 (1992): 203–243.

20. Fred C. Lunenburg, "Louder than Words: The Hidden Power of Nonverbal Communication in the Workplace," *International Journal of Scholarly Academic Intellectual Diversity* 12, no. 1 (2010): 1–5.

21. DePaulo, "Nonverbal Behavior and Self-Presentation."

22. Audrey Holland, ed., *34th Clinical Aphasiology Conference: A Special Issue of Aphasiology* (New York: Psychology Press, 2005).

23. Angela Fagerlin, Brian J. Zikmund-Fisher, and Peter A. Ubel, "Helping Patients Decide: Ten Steps to Better Risk Communication," *Journal of the National Cancer Institute* 103, no. 19 (2011): 1436–1443. doi: 10.1093/jnci/djr318.

24. Allan Paivio, *Mental Representations: A Dual Coding Approach* (New York: Oxford University Press, 1990).

25. Mark A. Staal, "Stress, Cognition, and Human Performance: A Literature Review and Conceptual Framework," Ames Research Center, Moffett Field, California. NASA/TM—2004–212824, 2004. http://human-factors.arc.nasa.gov/flightcognition/Publications/IH_054_Staal.pdf.

26. Goldberg, *Clinical Skills for Speech-Language Pathologists*.

27. Stacey T. Lutz and William G. Huitt, "Information Processing and Memory: Theory and Applications," *Educational Psychology Interactive* (Valdosta, GA: Valdosta State University, 2003). http://www.edpsycinteractive.org/papers/infoproc.pdf.

28. Jane Turner and Brian Kelly, "Emotional Dimensions of Chronic Disease, *Western Journal of Medicine* 172, no. 2 (2000): 124–128.

29. "Basic Facts About Hearing Loss," *Hearing Loss Association of America*, http://www.hearingloss.org/content/basic-facts-about-hearing-loss.

30. Geoffrey A. Kerchner et al., "Cognitive Processing Speed in Older Adults: Relationship with White Matter Integrity," *PLoS ONE* 7, no. 11 (2012): e50425.

31. Richard Culatta and Stanley A. Goldberg, *Stuttering Therapy: An Integrated Approach to Theory and Practice* (Boston: Allyn & Bacon, 1996).

32. Rodger E. Ziemer and William H. Tranter, *Principles of Communications: Systems Modulation and Noise*. 5th ed. (San Francisco: Wiley, 2001).

33. Ibid.

34. Ida Siveke et al., "Adaptation of Binaural Processing in the Adult Brainstem Induced by Ambient Noise," *The Journal of Neuroscience*, 32, no. 2 (2012): 462–473. doi: 10.1523/JNEUROSCI.2094-11.2012.

35. Ofer Zur, "Power in Psychotherapy and Counseling: Exploring the 'Inherent Power Differential' and Related Myths About Therapists' Omnipotence and Clients' Vulnerability," *Independent Practitioner* 29, no. 3 (2002): 160–164.

36. Richard Avedon, "Noto, Sicily" (1947), *Your Monkey Called*, April 14, 2009, http://yourmonkeycalled.com/post/96373884/richard-avedon-noto-sicily-1947-this-is.

CHAPTER 6

1. Andrew Rosenblum et al., "Opioids and the Treatment of Chronic Pain: Controversies, Current Status, and Future Directions," *Experimental and Clinical Psychopharmacology* 16, no. 5 (2008): 405–416. doi: 10.1037/a0013628.

2. C. Schneider, Steven H. Yale, and M. Larson, "Principles of Pain Management," *Clinical Medicine & Research* 1, no. 4 (2003): 337–340.

3. Nicola L. Lewis and John E. Williams, "Acute Pain Management in Patients Receiving Opioids for Chronic and Cancer Pain," *Continuing Education in Anaesthesia, Critical Care & Pain* 5, no. 4 (2005): 127–129. doi: 10.1093/bjaceaccp/mki034.

4. Mark J. Edlund et al., "Risk Factors for Clinically Recognized Opioid Abuse and Dependence Among Veterans Using Opioids for Chronic Non-Cancer Pain," *Pain* 129, no. 3 (2007): 355–362.

5. H. Breivik et al., "Assessment of Pain," *British Journal of Anaesthesia*, 101, no. 1 (2008): 17–24.

6. Inna Belfer, "The Nature of Nurture of Human Pain," *Scientifica* (2013), http://dx.doi.org/10.1155/2013/415279.

7. "Adult Cancer Pain," *National Comprehensive Cancer Network* (2013), http://oralcancerfoundation.org/treatment/pdf/pain.pdf.

8. Rod MacLeod, Jane Vella-Brincat, and Sandy Macleod, *The Palliative Care Handbook: Guidelines for Clinical Management and Symptom Control*. 7th ed. (Sydney, Australia: HammondPress, 2014).

9. Janice Reynolds, Debra Drew, and Colleen Dunwoody, "American Society for Pain Management Nursing Position Statement: Pain Management at the End of Life," August (2013). http://www.aspmn.org/documents/PainManagementattheEndofLife_August2013.pdf.

10. Marilyn J. Field and Christine K. Cassel, eds., *Approaching Death: Improving Care at the End of Life* (Washington, DC: National Academies Press, 1997): 6.

11. Ibid.

12. T. J. Cicero, J. A. Inciardi, and A. Munoz, "Trends in Abuse of Oxycontin and Other Opioid Analgesics in the United States: 2002-2004," *Journal of Pain* 6, no. 10 (2005): 662-672.

13. Rosenblum et al., "Opioids and the Treatment of Chronic Pain."

14. Ibid.

15. "Benefits of Mindfulness: Practices for Improving Emotional and Physical Well-Being," *Helpguide.org*, http://www.helpguide.org/harvard/benefits-of-mindfulness.htm.

16. Rosenblum et al., "Opioids and the Treatment of Chronic Pain."

17. Eric J. Cassell, "The Nature of Suffering and the Goals of Medicine," *New England Journal of Medicine* 306, no. 11 (1982): 639–645.

18. Carlo A. Porro et al., "Does Anticipation of Pain Affect Cortical Nociceptive Systems?" *The Journal of Neuroscience* 22, no. 8 (2002): 3206–3214.

19. Ibid.

20. David A. Seminowicz and Karen D. Davis, "Interactions of Pain Intensity and Cognitive Load: The Brain Stays on Task," *Cerebral Cortex* 17, no. 6 (2007): 1412–1422. doi: 10.1093/cercor/bhl052.

21. Christian Sprenger et al., "Attention Modulates Spinal Cord Responses to Pain," *Current Biology* 22, no. 11 (2012): 1019–1022. doi: 10.1016/jcub.2012.04.006.

22. Russell E. Hilliard, "Music Therapy in Hospice and Palliative Care: A Review of the Empirical Data," *Evidence-Based Complementary and Alternative Medicine* 2, no. 2 (2005): 173–178.

23. Clare C. O'Callaghan, "Pain, Music Creativity and Music Therapy in Palliative Care," *American Journal of Hospice & Palliative Care* 13, no. 2 (1996): 43–49.

24. Mimi Hanks-Bell, Kathleen Halvey, and Judith A. Paice, "Pain Assessment and Management in Aging," *The Online Journal of Issues in Nursing* 9, no. 3 (2004). http://www.nursingworld.org/MainMenuCategories/ANAMarketplace/ANAPeriodicals/OJIN/TableofContents/Volume92004/No3Sept04/ArticlePreviousTopic/PainAssessmentandManagementinAging.aspx. MainMenuCategories/

ANAMarketplace/ANAPeriodicals/OJIN/TableofContents/Volume92004/
No3Sept04/ArticlePreviousTopic/PainAssessmentandManagementinAging.aspx.

25. Rev. Master Jiyu-Kennett and Rev. Daizui MacPhillamy, *Roar of the Tigress: The Oral Teachings of Rev. Master Jiyu-Kennett, Western Woman and Zen Master* Vol. II. (Shasta, CA: Shasta Abbey Press, 2005).

26. Rick Warren, "The Purpose of Redemptive Suffering," *Daily Hope with Rick Warren*, http://rickwarren.org/devotional/english/the-purpose-of-redemptive-suffering.

CHAPTER 7

1. Michael T. Garrett, *Walking on the Wind: Cherokee Teachings for Harmony and Balance* (Rochester, VT: Bear & Company, 1998).

2. Ahmed Elsayem et al., "Use of Palliative Sedation for Intractable Symptoms in the Palliative Care Unit of a Comprehensive Cancer Center," *Supportive Care in Cancer* 17, no. 53 (2009): 59.

3. Eduardo Bruera, "Palliative Sedation: When and How?" *Journal of Clinical Oncology* 30, no. 12 (2012): 1258–1259. doi: 10.1200/JCO.2011.41.1223.

4. Marco Maltoni et al., "Palliative Sedation in End-of-Life Care and Survival: A Systematic Review," *Journal of Clinical Oncology* 30, no. 12 (2012): 1378–1383.

5. Stephen R. Connor and Maria Cecilia Sepulveda Bermedo, eds., *Global Atlas of Palliative Care at the End of Life*, Worldwide Palliative Care Alliance and World Health Organization (January 2014), http://www.who.int/nmh/Global_Atlas_of_Palliative_Care.pdf.

6. Sogyal Rinpoche, *The Tibetan Book of Living and Dying* (San Francisco: HarperCollins, 2012).

7. Joan K. Monin and Richard Schulz, "Interpersonal Effects of Suffering in Older Adult Caregiving Relationships," *Psychology and Aging* 24, no. 3 (2009): 681–695. doi: 10.1037/a0016355.

8. Personal communication during a workshop conducted by the Zen Hospice Center in San Francisco, California, in 2002.

9. Sogyal Rinpoche, *Glimpse After Glimpse: Daily Reflections on Living and Dying* (New York: HarperOne, 1995), October 3rd.

10. Lodovico Balducci, "Death and Dying: What the Patient Wants," *Annals of Oncology* 23, no. 3 (2012): 56–61. doi: 10.1093/annonc/mds089.

11. Robert Hurwitt, "Dean Goodman: Longtime Player in Bay Area Theater," *SF Gate*, July 6, (2006), http://www.sfgate.com/bayarea/article/Dean-Goodman-longtime-player-in-Bay-Area-2493327.php.

12. "Being With Someone When They Die," *Dying Matters*, http://www.dyingmatters.org/page/being-someone-when-they-die.

13. Cheryl Arenella, "Artificial Nutrition and Hydration at the End of Life: Beneficial or Harmful?" *American Hospice Foundation*, http://americanhospice

.org/caregiving/artificial-nutrition-and-hydration-at-the-end-of-life-beneficial-or-harmful/.

14. Barbara O'Brien, "The Wheel of Life: The Realm of Hungry Ghosts," *About.com*, http://buddhism.about.com/od/tibetandeities/ig/Wheel-of-Life-Gallery/Hungry-Ghosts-Realm.htm.

15. Christopher W. Kerr et al., "End-of-Life Dreams and Visions: A Longitudinal Study of Hospice Patients' Experiences. *Journal of Palliative Medicine* 17, no. 3 (2014): 296–303. doi: 10.1089/jpm.2013.0371.

16. Stan Goldberg, *Lessons for the Living: Stories of Forgiveness, Gratitude, and Courage at the End of Life* (Boston: Trumpeter, 2009).

17. Ibid.

18. Rinpoche, *Glimpse After Glimpse*.

19. Anonymous, "The Art of Dying Well," in *Medieval Popular Religion, 1000–1500, a Reader*. ed. John Shinners (London: Broadview Press, 1997), 525–535. English translation.

CHAPTER 8

1. William Shakespeare, *History of Richard II*, OpenSource Shakespeare, Act IV, Scene 1, http://www.opensourceshakespeare.org/views/plays/play_view.php?WorkID=richard2&Act=4&Scene=1&Scope=sceneh.

2. Herbert C. Kelman, "Interests, Relationships, Identities: Three Central Issues for Individuals and Groups in Negotiating Their Social Environment," *Annual Review of Psychology* 57 (2006): 1–26, doi: 10.1146/annurev.psych.57.102904.190156.

3. Thich Nhat Hanh, *The Path of Emancipation* (New Delhi: Full Circle Publishing, 2010).

4. Hirsch, Arnold R. *Making the Second Ghetto: Race and Housing in Chicago, 1940–1960*. (New York: Cambridge University Press, 1983).

5. Makoto Ueda, *Basho and His Interpreters* (Stanford, CA: Stanford University Press, 1995), 342.

6. David Schiller, ed., *The Little Zen Companion* (New York: Workman Publishing, 1994), 75.

7. Elizabeth Kübler-Ross and David Kessler, *On Grief and Grieving: Finding the Meaning of Grief Through the Five Stages of Loss* (New York: Scribner, 2014).

8. Abe Masao and Steven Heine, eds., *A Study of Dōgen: His Philosophy and Religion* (Albany, NY: SUNY Press, 1992).

9. Peter D. Cramer, *Listening to Prozac: The Landmark Book About Antidepressants and the Remaking of the Self*, rev. ed. (New York: Penguin Books, 1997).

10. John Lennon, *Double Fantasy Stripped Down* © 2010 Capitol. Compact disc.

11. Neville Goddard, *The Power of Awareness* (CreateSpace, 2013).

12. The Dalai Lama, *The Art of Happiness: A Handbook for Living*, 10th Anniversary ed. (New York: Riverhead, 2009).

13. Pema Chodron, *The Pocket Pema Chodron* (Boston: Shambhala Pocket Classics, 2008).

14. Stan Goldberg, "The 10 Rules of Change," *Psychology Today*. Last updated 12/4/12. https://www.psychologytoday.com/articles/200210/the-10-rules-change.

15. Ibid.

16. B. F. Skinner, *Science and Human Behavior* (New York: Free Press, 1965).

17. Mikhail Maiorov and Stefan Spinler, "Practical Framework for Intellectual Property Valuation," in *Intellectual Property in Academia: A Practical Guide for Scientists and Engineers*, ed. Nadya Reingand (Boca Raton, FL: CRC Press, 2011), 47.

18. Avi Karni et al., "The Acquisition of Skilled Motor Performance: Fast and Slow Experience-Driven Changes in Primary Motor Cortex, *Proceedings of the National Academy of Sciences* 95, no. 3 (1998): 861–868.

19. Gail B. Peterson, "A Day of Great Illumination: B. F. Skinner's Discovery of Shaping," *Journal of the Experimental Analysis of Behavior* 82, no. 3 (2004): 317–328.

20. Skinner, *Science and Human Behavior*.

21. Sean M. Bulger, Derek J. Mohr, and Richard T. Walls, "Stack the Deck in Favor of Your Students by Using the Four Aces of Effective Teaching," *Journal of Effective Teaching* 5, no. 2 (2002), http://uncw.edu/cte/et/articles/bulger/.

22. Alexandra Carter and Janet O'Shea, *The Routlege Dance Studies Reader* (New York: Routlege, 2010), 96.

23. K. Anders Ericsson, Ralf Th. Krampe, and Clemens Tesch-Romer, "The Role of Deliberate Practice in the Acquisition of Expert Performance," *Psychological Review* 100, no. 3 (1993): 363–406.

24. Jerry L. Deffenbacher and Richard M. Suinn, "Systematic Desensitization and the Reduction of Anxiety," *The Counseling Psychologist* 16, no. 1 (1998): 9–30.

25. Todd R. Schachtman and Steve S. Reilly, *Associative Learning and Conditioning Theory: Human and Non-Human Applications* (New York: Oxford University Press, 2011).

Appendix

WHAT TO DO FOR YOUR LOVED ONE AND HOW TO DO IT

CHAPTER 1: THE BASICS

Reduce The Chaos of Cancer

1. Expect a cancer journey to take an uncertain path.
2. Don't underestimate the psychological effects of uncertainty.

Assume The World of Your Loved One Differs From Yours

3. Don't allow your agenda to prevent the use of compassionate behaviors
4. Take the perspective of your loved one who is living with cancer
   rather than your own.
5. Don't evaluate a loved one using your perspective.

Honestly Express Your Feelings

6. Express your feelings about your loved one's cancer.
7. Don't expect your loved one to share her feelings if you can't share
   yours.
8. If you have difficulty expressing feelings, start with how children
   experience the world.
9. The past is the source of most defensive mechanisms—you don't
   need them in the present.

Change Compassionate Thoughts into Helpful Behaviors

10. Compassionate thoughts are not sufficient to be helpful. You need to transform them into behaviors.
11. You will need to understand your loved one's world before you can change compassionate thoughts into helpful behaviors.
12. Be prepared do acts displaying compassion.
13. Your compassion will be a gift to both you and your loved one.

Recognize Reactions to Cancer Differ

14. How your loved one reacts to emotional events is a blueprint for how she will respond to a diagnosis of cancer.
15. An emotional reaction to a cancer diagnosis by your loved one is better in the long run than a "stiff-upper-lip" attitude.
16. Accept your loved one's version of the facts instead of arguing about them.

Why It's Not a Battle

17. Don't compliment us on being survivors.
18. Compliment us on learning how to live with cancer.
19. Accept how your loved views her confrontation with cancer, regardless what you believe.
20. Focus on small winnable conflicts with cancer rather than ones involving survival.

What You Will Experience

21. You will experience feelings of helplessness.
22. You can place yourself in your loved one's shoes, but don't expect to get it completely right.
23. You are not God. You will make mistakes.
24. Don't feel guilty about satisfying your needs.

Thinking About Cancer is Not the Same as Experiencing It

25. Thinking about cancer will not give you the type of understanding derived from experiencing it.

Reduce Stress and Take Care of Your Needs

26. If you don't reduce stress, your ability to be compassionate and helpful will be reduced.
27. Although there are many ways of reducing stress, meditation can be used when the time is short and caregiving help is minimal or nonexistent.
28. Do a stress-reduction activity twice a day, for fifteen minutes if possible.

CHAPTER 2: REVEALING A CANCER DIAGNOSIS

The Decision to Reveal a Cancer Diagnosis

1. Saying "I have cancer" is an invitation to participate in what may be a long journey.
2. View the sharing of a cancer diagnosis as an honor.

Be Careful About Using Labels

3. Don't treat the person living with cancer as if he is the disease.

Be Supportive and Specific

4. Be specific regarding what you're offering to do.
5. Your loved one may be rejecting your help not because she doesn't need it but rather because accepting help acknowledges the effects of cancer.
6. Make a list of your loved one's daily activities. Then ask her for input on how you can help.
7. The repeated rejection of help may require a discussion of how the cancer is changing your loved one.
8. Cancer is dynamic, and what you got right today may be wrong tomorrow.
9. It's preferable to be overhelpful than to underestimate your loved one's needs.

Balance Hope With Reality

10. Don't be a cheerleader.
11. Limit hope to achievable goals.

12. Don't inundate your loved one with news of miracle cures.
13. Withhold your unqualified support for treatment protocols lacking data.
14. Support alternative approaches if the protocol isn't a substitution for one with data.
15. Visit FDA.com or other reputable websites if you think a treatment protocol is a scam or worthless.
16. Negotiate objective criteria for ending a treatment's use.

The Professional Management of Cancer

17. Honor your loved one's views regarding the reality of her prognosis.
18. Confine your optimism to the successful completion of small events, not the defeat of cancer.

Balancing Honesty With Compassion

19. Being helpful may involve living in the gray area of honesty.
20. Your primary goal is to be supportive, not to assume the role of a judge.

Build Trust Early

21. Establish trust well in advance of when you need it.
22. The development of trust is cumulative. Each trustworthy action moves it forward.
23. Trust is difficult if not impossible to regain after you lose it.
24. Develop trust by doing what you say you will do, listening compassionately without judging, witnessing your loved one's pain without withdrawing, and skillfully balancing honesty with support.

Send Good Thoughts

25. Sending good thoughts says to a person with cancer you care. It establishes a bond.
26. Good thoughts can be religious or secular.
27. Don't limit good thoughts to a cure.

Help the Person in Emotional Shock to Function

28. There is no specific amount of time emotional shock will last.
29. Emotional shock can lead to depression.

30. Don't rely on drugs to stop emotional shock; use supportive actions.
31. Reduce the number of nonmedical decisions, delay medical decisions when possible, and assist your loved one to understand the consequences of each choice.

Accept and Support Treatment Decisions

32. Support difficult choices even if you disagree.
33. Ask for an explanation if you don't understand why your loved one made a decision with which you disagree.
34. A choice to end life-extending treatment is not a reflection on you.

CHAPTER 3: A LIFE OF UNCERTAINTY

When You Become Collateral Damage

1. Treat cancer as a community event, not something owned by your loved one.
2. Much of what your loved one is feeling may be unshared.
3. Plan for instability rather than a predictable life.

How Side Effects Will Change Your Loved One's Life

4. Expect exhaustion from the effects of cancer and its treatment and side effects.
5. Accept the presence of treatment side effects ranging from mild to severe, none to many, those expected, and those not expected.
6. Reduce the number of scheduled social events.

The Meaning of Gratitude and Its Absence

7. Graciously accept gratitude as the expression of vulnerability.
8. Don't take personally a lack recognition for your efforts.
9. Treat a lack of gratitude as a signal it's time to discuss resistance to increased dependence.

Be Supportive as Examination Appointments Approach

10. Take on additional responsibilities as the appointment date nears.
11. Be supportive of what your loved one is experiencing rather than exhibiting unbridled optimism regarding the checkup's outcome.

Help Create Simplicity, Stability, and Control

12. Strive to simplify your and your loved one's life.
13. Accept behaviors that enhance your loved one's sense of stability and control.
14. Introduce predictability.
15. Help organize your loved one's life.
16. Prioritize what's important for the cancer journey; then act on it.

Insist on Treatment With Dignity

17. Insist that your loved one is more than a "cancer patient" or a medical lesson.
18. Accept your loved one's designation of what's dignified.
19. Always ask whether what you think should occur is acceptable to her.

Balance Independence and Dependence

20. Ask your loved one whether she needs assistance before providing it.
21. Assume the balance between independence and assistance continually shifts.
22. It's better to be overly helpful rather than not helpful enough.
23. As independence declines, reinforce it, even if it involves inconsequential behaviors.
24. Help your loved one let go of parts of her identity that no longer exist.

Look for the Lost Emotions Behind Grief

25. Don't try to replace the lost ability or activity. Rather, help your loved one find activities to regenerate the emotions.
26. Grief doesn't have a timetable or steps taking you from despair to joy.
27. Help your loved one shift the focus from unobtainable goals to smaller achievable ones.

Don't Assume Your Loved One is Aware of Interpersonal Problems

28. Don't confront your loved one when the unskillful words or behaviors are occurring. Do it when they cease.

29. Confine your feedback to facts and how you felt when you explain the effects of hurtful behaviors and words. Don't frame the discussion as "this is what you did wrong."
30. Use code phrases as a shortcut feedback approach.
31. Accept a loved one's apology for inappropriate words or behaviors without being judgmental.

Thinking is Not the Key to Happiness

32. Don't try to increase your loved one's happiness by talking or thinking.
33. Help your loved one find three positive things to do every day.
34. Rely on your loved one's passion for selecting positive activities.
35. Help your loved one stop doing negative things and replace them with positive ones.
36. Make change almost as easy as not changing.

CHAPTER 4: THE NATURE OF LOSSES

Losses Are a Part of Life

1. Accept the changes in your loved one's personality because of a significant loss.
2. Don't use the "glass is half full" argument.

Losing What Gives Joy

3. Expect changes in your loved one's behaviors if the losses are significant.

Anger

4. Expect your loved one's anger to spill into areas not related to his losses.
5. The anger expressed can be generated internally and through external reactions to the loss.
6. Expect anger to distort reality.
7. Don't marginalize your loved one's anger or take it personally.

Distortions

8. Expect to see distortions

Don't Fill Up Time

9. Don't search for "time fillers." Rather, find activities appropriate to your loved one's new identity.

Expectations Following Losses

10. Don't expect your loved one to act as he did before the loss of a significant ability or activity.
11. Base expectations on your loved one's new identity, not on one that no longer exists.

Accept Reordering of Priorities

12. Don't assume that what was important before the diagnosis is still important and vice versa.
13. Adjust your behaviors and expectations to the new context.

The Bigger Picture

14. Don't ignore the big picture when you try to understand your loved one's behaviors.
15. Assume that a behavior appears strange because you don't understand its meaning.
16. Don't use the context of a healthy person to understand the decisions of a person living with cancer.
17. Search for how the hidden meaning of behaviors is related to issues of closure.
18. Don't judge behaviors within a vacuum. Always assume they connect to the past.

Accept Changes in Identity

19. Changes in identity affect perceptions and behaviors.
20. Reassure your loved one of your continued support without minimizing the effects of cancer.
21. Changes in identity may not be stable. Identities change as losses accumulate.
22. Help your loved one adjust to her new identity rather than maintaining she's the same person she was before the diagnosis.
23. Think of cancer as a subtractive process.

CHAPTER 5: CONVERSATIONS

Why and How to Analyze Conversations

1. A conversational analysis will enable you to understand how the style of your interaction affects your loved one.
2. Don't be concerned about the sophistication of your analysis. Simple is better than sophisticated and some is better than none.
3. Your analysis of the conversation can be short since there is consistency in how we communicate. A ten-minute sample is sufficient.

Listen More and Talk Less

4. Sometimes compassionate listening is more supportive than filling the silence with words.
5. Allow silence to be the breathing space in which your loved one prepares to share painful feelings or topics.
6. Don't interrupt and do be nonjudgmental.

Assure Conversational Flow

7. Connect your comments directly to those of your loved one.
8. Be prepared to follow the conversation's trend.
9. Identify the type of statements moving a conversation forward and ones impeding it.
10. Use dialogues rather than successive monologues to develop bonding.
11. Allow your loved one to speak as much or more than you do.
12. Engage more in conversations and less in question-and-answer interactions.
13. If you are using a question format, try to keep the questions open ended rather than closed.

Clearly Express Ideas

14. Intonation will be used to determine your feelings if your words and intonation don't match.
15. Discuss your concerns instead of hiding your feelings by monitoring your intonation, since hiding the discrepancy will most likely be unsuccessful.
16. Use simple grammatical structures and words even if your loved one's cognitive ability is normal.

17. Minimize the number of ideas within each phrase for important issues

18. Compensate for the effects of drugs, medications, and emotional problems by slowing speech, but not to where it sounds abnormal.

19. Your choice of words should account for your loved one's physical and emotional needs.

Prevent Message Interference

20. Minimize noise.
21. Don't use noise for distraction.
22. Always turn off all media during important conversations.
23. Your loved one's insistence that a noise source remains can be an indication she fears dealing with the topic or wants to mute her feelings.

The Importance of Timing

24. Don't force difficult discussions. Wait until your loved one is ready.

Look for Hidden Meanings

25. Don't speculate on the hidden meaning. Explain to your loved one you need more clarification

CHAPTER 6: DISCOMFORT, PAIN, AND SUFFERING

Medication

1. Accept a loved one's decision to start with the maximum prescribed dosage.
2. Addiction rarely occurs in the management of cancer-related pain.
3. Use a hospital-based 0–10 pain management continuum and accept the number your loved one provides.
4. Track the increase or decrease of pain using the 0–10 continuum.

Treating Discomfort

5. Mild long-term discomfort can have the same psychological effect as chronic pain.

6. Opiates are abused to reduce the psychological effects of discomfort.
7. Accept the legitimacy of discomfort as a debilitating condition requiring nondrug methods.

Treating Chronic Pain

8. Don't expect long-term relief from mind control.
9. Chronic pain will affect everything your loved one experiences.
10. The occurrence of chronic pain is not predictable.

Reducing Suffering

11. Differentiate pain from suffering.
12. Suffering can be emotional or physical.
13. You will want to stop the suffering but may be limited to compassionate witnessing.

The Boundaries of Pain are Porous

14. Treatment of pain goes beyond its beginning and end points.
15. Expect pain to affect your loved one's activities even when it's absent.
16. Discuss with your loved one what you can do to restructure her environment to reduce the pain.

Thinking During Pain

17. Don't expect clarity of thought when your loved one is experiencing intense pain.

Use Distraction to Minimize Pain

18. Distractions may minimize pain but not eliminate it.
19. Find activities that require minimal concentration.
20. Use the following principles if you play live or recorded music: play softly, keep the transitions between notes small, and look for songs starting with low notes and ending with higher ones.
21. Distracting activities should not require much thought, should pull your loved one forward, and should be positive enough to affect the negativity of the pain.

Accept Sudden Changes in Plans

22. Changes in plans and cancellations often are caused by more than one problem.
23. Expect hope at being able to attend an event to exceed her physical or emotional ability.
24. If your loved one cancels an event, offer to stay with her despite her insistence you go by yourself.
25. Schedule visits and possible events even if your loved one anticipates the presence of pain.
26. Acknowledge the legitimacy of your loved one's reasons for canceling.

Don't Romanticize Pain

27. Don't try to convince your loved one she can learn anything from pain—especially when it is occurring.
28. Listen without being judgmental if a loved one wants to talk about the lessons she has gained from pain.

Witnessing Pain

29. Hold your loved one's hand when he is experiencing pain.
30. Always ask your loved one what you can do as he experiences pain.
31. Don't feel guilty if you're not capable of witnessing intense pain.

CHAPTER 7: EASING A LOVED ONE'S DEATH

Support End-of-Life Decisions

1. Support your loved one's decision to stop life-extending treatment even if you disagree.
2. Supporting your loved one's decision to stop life-extending treatment is only the first step in your support.
3. The reasons for stopping life-extending treatment can be based either on physical or psychological suffering.

Support Unrealistic Beliefs When It's Compassionate

4. It's more compassionate to be complicit in a delusion rather than to crushing a person's hope, even if you think her beliefs are unrealistic.

5. Your nonconfrontive position may lead to your loved one's accepting her terminal condition.

When to Begin Discussing Hospice

6. Become knowledgeable about hospice services as soon as possible.
7. Begin exploring hospice immediately after the terminal prognosis if your loved one will accept it.
8. Don't start the discussion of hospice if your loved one does not accept the terminal diagnosis. Wait until she initiates the conversation.
9. Visit freestanding hospices and organizations providing in-home services with your loved one.

Help Your Loved One Let Go

10. Helping your loved one let go of life is dependent on your ability to let go of her.
11. Move your loved one's fixating on past lapses in judgment to the present by highlighting the positive effects her life had on you and others.
12. If your loved one expresses the loss of the future, convince her of the legacy she leaves.

Expect Helplessness

13. Realize that your goal is not to save your loved one, but to serve her as she dies.

Dying is Hard Work

14. Approach dying as a process rather than as an event with clear beginning and end points.
15. Expect long-term exhaustion and short-lived euphoria.
16. The hard work of dying involves both the body and the mind.

Don't be Afraid to Talk About Death

17. Don't spend time searching for the right words. Speak from your heart and you'll be fine.
18. Don't initiate a conversation about dying if your loved one isn't ready. Wait until she initiates it.

19. Allow periods of silence to be the preparation your loved one needs to talk about his death.

Don't Assume Spirituality and Religion are Enough

20. Neither spirituality nor religion by itself may be enough to ease a loved one's death.
21. Regardless of your loved one's spirituality or religious convictions, search for any unfinished business that might be making the transition more difficult.
22. Don't attempt a deathbed conversion. Efforts generate more annoyance than creation of states of grace.
23. Honor your loved one's beliefs regardless how much you believe they will result in terrible afterlife consequences.

Asking for Forgiveness

24. If your loved one asks for forgiveness, grant it, without qualifications or lengthy rebuttals.
25. Create substitute forms of forgiveness if your loved one can't be forgiven by the offended person.
26. Forgive your loved one when she asks for it, even if you don't think she did anything that requires forgiveness.

Help Tie Up Loose Ends

27. Don't dismiss the need for completing unfinished business.
28. Some efforts to "clean one's plate" before dying are literal, while others are allegorical.
29. Participate in any attempts that seem related to finishing something.

Saying and Accepting Thanks

30. Help your loved one complete unfinished tasks.
31. Accept all expressions of gratitude even if you think that what you did was inconsequential.
32. Host a good-bye party.
33. Encourage your loved one's family and friends to publically express thanks for all she contributed to them.

Don't Grieve Excessively in Your Loved One's Presence

34. The excessive display of grief in front of your loved one can prolong her dying.
35. Assume that your loved one can hear you even if she is in a coma since hearing is one of the last senses to leave.

Don't Force Food or Water

36. Don't force your loved one to ingest either food or liquids if her body is shutting down.
37. Don't expect death to occur soon after food and fluids are stopped.
38. Use a sponge paddle to alleviate dryness in the mouth or on the lips.

Give Legitimacy to Private Experiences

39. Accept your loved one's private experiences if they are uplifting.
40. Don't interpret uplifting private experiences.
41. Help your loved one dismiss frightening visions through objective means rather than words.

Give Permission to Die

42. Your final gift to your loved one will be permission to die.
43. Use simple words and only state the offer once or, if you believe your loved one didn't comprehend what you said, a few times more.
44. Loved ones may be able to "schedule" their death.
45. Your loved one's dying when you leave the room is more an act of love than a statement of anything negative about your relationship.

How to Create a Vigil

46. Remove objects associated with the disease or its treatment.
47. Fill the room with objects, music, and smells having a positive connection with your loved one's life.
48. Ask the hospice volunteer to be responsible for the vigil if you are uncomfortable managing it.

49. A vigil will ease your loved one's death and create positive memories for you.

What to Do When Death is Imminent

50. No words can describe what you will feel at the death of your loved one.
51. Listen to and observe what is happening to your loved one before you act.
52. Rely on your loved one's history to find words and behaviors to ease her death.

What to Do After the Moment of Death

53. Sit and do nothing.
54. Reflect on your loved one's life and the impact she had on you.
55. Create a ritual.
56. Ceremoniously clean and prepare your loved one's body.

You Did the Best You Could

57. The demands on you may be greater than your ability to fulfill them.
58. You did the best you could given the circumstances of your life.

Lessons You Will Learn

59. You will receive gems of wisdom from participating in a loved one's death.
60. Don't try to understand the lessons when they are occurring. It may take months or years for you to appreciate them.

CHAPTER 8: RECOVERING JOY

Understanding Grief's Intensity

1. There is no hierarchy for sorrow.
2. The more dependent a relationship with a lost loved one, the greater the grief.
3. The ending of a troubling relationship has the same effects on identity as the loss of a positive and loving one.

Acceptance and Moving Forward

4. You'll need to accept your loss before you can move forward.
5. Shift your focus from the loss to what you wish to regain.

Therapy: How Much Time to Grieve?

6. Don't expect rigid timelines for grief.
7. Don't use "steps" as an accurate way of determining where you are in the grief process.
8. Whatever approach to grief reduction you choose, account for the effect of time on the development of long-term depression.

Living in the Present

9. Shift your awareness from the past and future to the present.
10. Your awareness should focus on identifying skills, activities, and people having the potential for generating the emotions you no longer have.

It Takes Energy to be Miserable

11. Take frequent breaks from your grief by focusing on something simple and concrete.

Finding the Lost Emotion

12. Choose one emotion for recovery that poses the least difficulties.
13. Don't confine your search to people. Skills and activities can also generate the lost emotion.
14. Don't assume that regaining one feeling will lead to recovering other emotions.
15. Be specific regarding the emotions you want to recover.

Universal Principles for Resurrecting Joy

16. Don't keep reaching for the "brass ring." You'll fail more than you'll succeed.
17. The completion of each small goal becomes the stepping-stone to your next objective.

18. Assume that the emotion you are trying to resurrect is complex.
19. Since change is frightening, do whatever is necessary to reduce the discomfort, including selecting smaller and more realistic goals.
20. Whatever you want to change should result in a positive outcome. If it does not, the new behavior or attitude will disappear.
21. Change should be almost as easy as not changing.
22. For change to be long lasting, it should be developed slowly.
23. The more you know about the principles of change, the more likely you will be successful.
24. Your attempts to recover an emotion should be structured.
25. If the new emotion is to become stable, it requires practice.
26. Develop associations for the resurrected emotions.
27. Striving for many small successes is better than continually failing by looking for only "big" successes.

Troubleshooting

28. Don't blame yourself for failures. Failures are opportunities to learn.
29. You will always be in transition

BIBLIOGRAPHY

Adler, Nancy E. and Ann E. K. Page, eds. *Cancer Care for the Whole Patient: Meeting Psychosocial Health Needs*. Washington, DC: National Academies Press, 2008.

"Adult cancer pain." *National Comprehensive Cancer Network* (2013). http://oral cancerfoundation.org/treatment/pdf/pain.pdf.

Alter, Adam. "Why It's Dangerous to Label People." *Psychology Today*, May 17 (2010). https://www.psychologytoday.com/blog/alternative-truths/201005/why-its-dangerous-label-people.

Anonymous. "The Art of Dying Well." In *Medieval Popular Religion, 1000–1500, A Reader*, edited by John Shinners, 525–535. London: Broadview Press, 1997. English translation.

Arenella, Cheryl. "Artificial Nutrition and Hydration at the End of Life: Beneficial or Harmful?" *American Hospice Foundation*. http://americanhospice.org/caregiving/artificial-nutrition-and-hydration-at-the-end-of-life-beneficial-or-harmful/.

Avedon, Richard. "Noto, Sicily" (1947). *Your Monkey Called*. April 14, 2009. http://yourmonkeycalled.com/post/96373884/richard-avedon-noto-sicily-1947-this-is.

Back, Anthony L., Susan M. Bauer-Wu, Cynda H. Rushton, and Joan Halifax. "Compassionate Silence in the Patient-Clinician Encounter: A Contemplative Approach." *Journal of Palliative Medicine* 12, no. 12 (2009): 1113–1117. doi: 10.1089/jpm.2009.0175.

Balducci, Lodovico. "Death and Dying: What the Patient Wants." *Annals of Oncology* 23, no. 3 (2012): 56–61. doi: 10.1093/annonc/mds089.

"Basic Facts About Hearing Loss." *Hearing Loss Association of America*. http://www.hearingloss.org/content/basic-facts-about-hearing-loss.

Bazzon, A., Andrew B. Newberg, William C. Cho, and Daniel A. Monti. "Diet and Nutrition in Cancer Survivorship and Palliative Care." *Evidence-Based Complementary and Alternative Medicine Volume 2013*. http://dx.doi.org/10.1155/2013/917647.

Beck, Lewis White, ed. *Eighteenth-Century Philosophy: Readings in the History of Philosophy*. New York: Free Press, 1966.

"Being With Someone When They Die," *Dying Matters*, http://www.dyingmatters.org/page/being-someone-when-they-die.

Belfer, Inna. "Nature and Nurture of Human Pain." *Scientifica* (2013). http://dx.doi.org/10.1155/2013/415279.

"Benefits of Mindfulness: Practices for Improving Emotional and Physical Well-Being." *Helpguide.org*. http://www.helpguide.org/harvard/benefits-of-mindfulness.htm.

Berlin, Heather A., and Christof Koch. "Defense Mechanisms: Neuroscience Meets Psychoanalysis." *Scientific American* April 1, 2009. http://www.scientificamerican.com/article/neuroscience-meets-psychoanalysis/.

Breivik, H., P. C. Borchgrevink, S. M. Allen, L. A. Rosseland, L. Romundstad, E. K. Hals, G. Kvarstein, and A. Stubhaug. "Assessment of pain." *British Journal of Anaesthesia* 101, no. 1 (2008): 17–24.

Bronowski, Jacob. *The Ascent of Man*. Boston: Brown, 1974.

Bruera, Eduardo. "Palliative Sedation: When and How?" *Journal of Clinical Oncology* 30, no. 12 (2012): 1258–1259. doi: 10.1200/JCO.2011.41.1223.

Bulger, Sean M., Derek J. Mohr, and Richard T. Walls. "Stack the Deck in Favor of Your Students by Using the Four Aces of Effective Teaching." *Journal of Effective Teaching* 5, no. 2 (2002). http://uncw.edu/cte/et/articles/bulger/.

Burns, David D. *The Feeling Good Handbook*. New York: Plume, 1999.

Cameron, Deborah. *Working with Spoken Discourse*. London: SAGE, 2001.

"Cancer Statistics." *National Cancer Institute*. 2015. http://www.cancer.gov/about-cancer/what-is-cancer/statistics.

"Cancer Treatment & Survivorship Facts & Figures." *American Cancer Society*. 2015. http://www.cancer.org/research/cancerfactsstatistics/survivor-facts-figures.

Cardoso, F., N. Harbeck, L. Fallowfield, S. Kyriakides, and E. Senkus. "Locally Recurrent or Metastatic Breast Cancer: ESMO Clinical Practice Guidelines for Diagnosis, Treatment and Follow-Up." *Annuals of Oncology* 23, no. 7 (2012): 11–19. doi: 10.1093/annonc/mds232.

Carroll, John B., ed. *Language, Thought, and Reality: Selected Writings of Benjamin Lee Whorf*. Boston: MIT Press, 1964.

Carter, Alexandra and Janet O'Shea. *The Routlege Dance Studies Reader*. New York: Routlege, 2010: 96.

Cassell, Eric J. "The Nature of Suffering and the Goals of Medicine." *New England Journal of Medicine* 306, no. 11 (1982): 639–645.

Castaneda, Carlos. *The Teachings of Don Juan: A Yaqui Way of Knowledge*. New York: Washington Square Press, 1985.

Centena, A. and G. Onik. *Prostate Cancer: A Patient's Guide to Treatment*. Omaha, NE: Addicus Books, 2014.

Chavan, Y. *Meditation for Beginners: How to Relieve Stress, Anxiety and Depression and Return to a State of Inner Peace and Happiness*. CreateSpace, 2014.

Chodron, Pema. *The Pocket Pema Chodron*. Boston: Shambhala Pocket Classics, 2008.

Cicero, T. J., J. A. Inciardi, and A. Munoz. "Trends in Abuse of Oxycontin and Other Opioid Analgesics in the United States: 2002-2004." *The Journal of Pain* 6, no. 10 (2005): 662–672.

Cline, D., O. John Ma, Rita Cydulka, Garth Meckler, Stephen Thomas, and Dan Handel. *Tintinalli's Emergency Medicine Manual*. 7th ed. Boston: McGraw-Hill, 2012.

Connor, Stephen R. and Maria Cecilia Sepulveda Bermedo, eds. *Global Atlas of Palliative Care at the End of Life*. Worldwide Palliative Care Alliance and World Health Organization (January 2014). http://www.who.int/nmh/Global_Atlas_of_Palliative_Care.pdf.

Cramer, Peter D. *Listening to Prozac: The Landmark Book About Antidepressants and the Remaking of the Self*. Rev. ed. New York: Penguin Books, 1997.

Culatta, Richard and Stanley A. Goldberg. *Stuttering Therapy: An Integrated Approach to Theory and Practice*. Boston: Allyn & Bacon, 1996.

Cunha, John P., ed. "Femara Side Effects Center." *RxList: The Internet Drug Index*. Last updated 5/22/15. http://www.rxlist.com/femara-side-effects-drug-center.htm.

D'Amico, Thomas A. "Outcomes After Surgery for Esophageal Cancer." *Gastrointestinal Cancer Research* 1, no. 5 (2007): 188–196.

Daugherty, Christopher K. and Fay J. Hlubocky. "What Are Terminally Ill Cancer Patients Told About Their Expected Deaths? A Study of Cancer Physicians' Self-Reports of Prognosis Disclosure." *Journal of Clinical Oncology* 26, no. 36 (2008): 5988–5993. doi: 10.1200/JCO.2008.17.2221.

Deb, Dhruba. "Understanding the Unpredictability of Cancer Using Chaos Theory and Modern Art Techniques." *Leonardo* 49, no. 1 (2016): 66–67. doi: 10.1162/LEON_a_01099.

Deffenbacher, Jerry L. and Richard M. Suinn. "Systematic Desensitization and the Reduction of Anxiety." *The Counseling Psychologist* 16, no. 1 (1988): 9–30.

DelVecchio, Rick. "Witness to Death's Spirituality." *Catholic San Francisco* July 8, 2009. http://www.catholic-sf.org/news_select.php?newsid=23&id=56182.

DePaulo, Bella M. "Nonverbal Behavior and Self-Presentation." *Psychological Bulletin* 111, no. 2 (1992): 203–243.

"Depression." *National Cancer Institute*. http://www.cancer.gov/about-cancer/coping/feelings/depression-pdq-section/all.

Edlund, Mark J., Diane Steffick, Teresa Hudsona, Katherine M. Harris, and Mark Sullivane. "Risk Factors for Clinically Recognized Opioid Abuse and Dependence Among Veterans Using Opioids for Chronic Non-Cancer Pain." *Pain* 129, no. 3 (2007): 355–362.

Elsayem Ahmed, Eardie Curry III, Jeanette Boohene, Mark F. Munsell, Bianca Calderon, Frank Hung, and Eduardo Bruera. "Use of Palliative Sedation for Intractable Symptoms in the Palliative Care Unit of a Comprehensive Cancer Center." *Supportive Care in Cancer* 17, no. 53 (2009): 59.

Ephratt, Michal. "The Functions of Silence." *Journal of Pragmatics* 40 (2008): 1909–1938. http://www.gloriacappelli.it/wp-content/uploads/2009/05/silence.pdf.

Ericsson, K. Anders, Ralf Th. Krampe, and Clemens Tesch-Romer. "The Role of Deliberate Practice in the Acquisition of Expert Performance." *Psychological Review* 100, no. 3 (1993): 363–406. https://www.nytimes.com/images/blogs/freakonomics/pdf/DeliberatePractice(PsychologicalReview).pdf.

Erlewine, Stephen Thomas. "Song Review by Stephen Thomas Erlewine." *AllMusic.* http://www.allmusic.com/song/bright-mississippi-mt0003455227.

Fagerlin, Angela, Brian J. Zikmund-Fisher, and Peter A. Ubel. "Helping Patients Decide: Ten Steps to Better Risk Communication." *Journal of the National Cancer Institute* 103, no. 19 (2011): 1436–1443. doi: 10.1093/jnci/djr318.

Falvo, Donna. *Medical and Psychosocial Aspects of Chronic Illness and Disability.* 5th ed. Burlington, MA: Jones & Bartlett Learning, 2013.

Ferrata, Paolo, Serafino Carta, Mattia Fortina, Daniele Scipio, Alberto Riva, and Salvatore Di Giacinto. "Painful Hip Arthroplasty: Definition." *Clinical Cases in Mineral and Bone Metabolism* 8, no. 2 (2011): 19–22.

Field, Marilyn J. and Christine K. Cassel, eds. *Approaching Death: Improving Care at the End of Life.* Washington, DC: National Academies Press, 1997.

Foote, R. et al. "The Clinical Case for Proton Beam Therapy." *Radiation Oncology* 7 (2012): 174. doi: 10.1186/1748-717X-7-174.

Frank, Mark G., Andreas Maroulis, and Darrin J. Griffin. "The Voice." In *Nonverbal Communication: Science and Applications*, edited by David Matsumoto, Mark Frank, and Hyi Sung Hwan, 53–74. Thousand Oaks, CA: SAGE, 2013.

Garrett, Michael T. *Walking on the Wind: Cherokee Teachings for Harmony and Balance.* Rochester, VT: Bear & Company, 1998.

Ginestier, P. *Anouilh.* Paris: Seghers, 1974.

Goddard, Neville. *The Power of Awareness.* CreateSpace, 2013.

Goldbach, P. "Decision Making by Patients and Physicians Together." *Health Affairs* 31, no. 8 (2012): 1909.

Goldberg, S. "Being Present at the Bedside." In *Communication and Positive Counseling*, edited by A. Holland. San Diego: Plural Publications, 2007.

Goldberg, Stan. "How Can I Be a Compassionate Caregiver?" *Buddhadharma* Winter (2011): 64–68.

———. *Leaning into Sharp Points: Practical Guidance and Nurturing Support for Caregivers.* Novato, CA: New World Library, 2012.

———. "Learning From Our Losses." *Living with Loss Magazine* 24, no. 4 (2009): 36–37.

———. *Lessons for the Living: Stories of Forgiveness, Gratitude, and Courage at the End of Life.* Boston: Trumpeter, 2013.

———. "Now the Bad News: Living with Chronic Illness." *Shambhala Sun Magazine* July (2013): 47–48.

———. *Ready to Learn: How to Help Your Preschooler Succeed.* New York: Oxford University Press, 2005.

———. "Shedding Your Fears: Bedside Etiquette for Dying Patients." *Topics in Stroke Rehabilitation* 13, no. 1 (2006): 63–67.

———. "The 10 Rules of Change." *Psychology Today.* Last updated 12/4/12. https://www.psychologytoday.com/articles/200210/the-10-rules-change.

———. "The Hard Work of Dying." *Shambhala Sun* November (2009): 27–29.

———. "Understanding Patients' Behaviors." *Hospice Volunteer News*, 3rd quarter (2009).

———. "Welcome to Kauai: What's That Strange Stick in Your Hand?" *Saltwater Fly Fishing* December (1999): 22–27.

———. "What Makes You Think You'll Live Forever?" *Buddhadharma* Fall (2010): 69–71.

———. "When You Can't Let Go." *stangoldbergwriter.com.* http://stangoldberg writer.com/about/when-you-cant-let-go/.

Goldberg, Stanley A. *Clinical Intervention: A Philosophy and Methodology for Clinical Practice.* New York: Macmillan, 1993.

———. *Clinical Skills for Speech-Language Pathologists: Practical Applications.* San Diego: Singular Press, 1996.

Greenberg, Neil, James A. Carr, and Cliff H. Summers. "Causes and Consequences of Stress." *Integrative & Comparative Biology* 42, no. 3 (2002): 508–516. doi: 10.1093/icb/42.3.508.

Hackworth, Martin. "The Physics of Motorcycles." *Motorcyclejazz.com.* http://www .motorcyclejazz.com/motorcycle_physics.htm.

Hancock, Karen, Josephine M. Clayton, Sharon M. Parker, Sharon Walder, Phyllis N. Butow, David Currow, Davina Ghersi, Paul Glare, and Rebecca Hagerty. "Truth-Telling in Discussing Prognosis in Advanced Life-Limiting Illnesses: A Systematic Review." *Palliative Medicine* 21 (2007): 507–517.

Hanks-Bell, Mimi, Kathleen Halvey, and Judith A. Paice. "Pain Assessment and Management in Aging." *The Online Journal of Issues in Nursing* 9, no. 3 (2004). http://www.nursingworld.org/MainMenuCategories/ANAMarketplace/ANA Periodicals/OJIN/TableofContents/Volume92004/No3Sept04/ArticlePrevi ousTopic/PainAssessmentandManagementinAging.aspx.

Hilliard, Russell E. "Music Therapy in Hospice and Palliative Care: A Review of the Empirical Data." *Evidence-Based Complementary and Alternative Medicine* 2, no. 2 (2005): 173–178.

Hirsch, Arnold R. *Making the Second Ghetto: Race and Housing in Chicago, 1940–1960.* New York: Cambridge University Press, 1983.

Hofman, M., J. L. Ryan, C. D. Figueroa-Moseley, P. Jean-Pierre, and G. R. Morrow. "Cancer-Related Fatigue: The Scale of the Problem." *The Oncologist* 12 Supplement 1 (2007): 4–10.

Holland, Audrey, ed. *34th Clinical Aphasiology Conference: A Special Issue of Aphasiology.* New York: Psychology Press, 2005.

Howlander, N. et al., eds. "SEER Cancer Statistics Review (CSR) 1975–2012." *National Cancer Institute.* Last updated 11/18/15. http://seer.cancer.gov/ csr/1975_2012/.

Hurwitt, Robert. "Dean Goodman: Longtime Player in Bay Area Theater." *SF Gate*. July 6 (2006). http://www.sfgate.com/bayarea/article/Dean-Goodman-longtime-player-in-Bay-Area-2493327.php.

Isaacson, Walter. *Steve Jobs*. New York: Simon & Schuster, 2015.

Jiyu-Kennett, Rev. Master, and Rev. Daizui MacPhillamy. *Roar of the Tigress: The Oral Teachings of Rev. Master Jiyu-Kennett, Western Woman and Zen Master*. Vol. II. Shasta, CA: Shasta Abbey Press, 2005.

Karatzanis, Alexander D., Georgios Psychogios, Frank Waldfahrer, Markus Kapsreiter, Johannes Zenk, George A. Velegrakis, and Heinrich Iro. "Management of Locally Advanced Laryngeal Cancer." *Journal of Otolaryngology-Head & Neck Surgery* 43 (2014): 4. doi: 10.1186/1916-0216-43-4.

Karni, Avi, Gundela Meyer, Christine Rey-Hipolito, Peter Jezzard, Michelle M. Adams, Robert Turner, and Leslie G. Ungerleider. "The Acquisition of Skilled Motor Performance: Fast and Slow Experience-Driven Changes in Primary Motor Cortex. *Proceedings of the National Academy of Sciences* 95, no. 3 (1998): 861–868.

Kelman, Herbert C. "Interests, Relationships, Identities: Three Central Issues for Individuals and Groups in Negotiating Their Social Environment." *Annual Review of Psychology* 57 (2006): 1–26. doi: 10.1146/annurev.psych.57.102904.190156.

Kerchner, Geoffrey A., Caroline A. Racine, Sandra Hale, Reva Wilheim, Victor Laluz, Bruce L. Miller, and Joel H. Kramer. "Cognitive Processing Speed in Older Adults: Relationship with White Matter Integrity." *PLoS ONE* 7, no. 11 (2012): e50425.

Kerr, Christopher W., James P. Donnelly, Scott T. Wright, Sarah M. Kuszczak, Anne Banas, Pei C. Grant, and Debra L. Luczkiewicz. "End-of-Life Dreams and Visions: A Longitudinal Study of Hospice Patients' Experiences." *Journal of Palliative Medicine* 17, no. 3 (2014): 296–303. doi: 10.1089/jpm.2013.0371.

Kind, Vicki. *The Caregiver's Path to Compassionate Decision Making: Making Choices for Those Who Can't*. Austin, TX: Greenleaf Book Group, 2010.

Knapp, Sarah, Allison Marziliano, and Anne Moyer. "Identity Threat and Stigma in Cancer Patients." *Health Psychology Open* 1, no. 1 (2014). doi: 10.1177/2055102914552281.

Korzybski, Alfred. *Science and Sanity: An Introduction to Non-Aristotelian Systems and General Semantics*. 5th ed. New York: Institute of General Semantics, 1995.

Koudenburg, Namkje, Tom Postmes, and Ernestine H. Gordijn. "Conversational Flow Promotes Solidarity." *PLoS ONE* 8, no. 11 (2013): e78363. doi: 10.1371/journal.pone.0078363.

Kübler-Ross, Elizabeth and David Kessler. *On Grief and Grieving: Finding the Meaning of Grief Through the Five Stages of Loss*. New York: Scribner, 2014.

Kumar, Ravi J., Al Barqawi, and E. David Crawford. "Adverse Events Associated with Hormonal Therapy for Prostate Cancer." *Reviews in Urology* 7, no. 5 (2005): S37–S43.

Lattman, Peter. "The Origins of Justice Stewart's 'I Know It When I See It.'" *Law-Blog at The Wall Street Journal Online* (September 27, 2007). http://blogs.wsj.com/law/2007/09/27/the-origins-of-justice-stewarts-i-know-it-when-i-see-it/.

Lawson, Karen and Sue Towey. "What Lifestyle Changes Are Recommended for Anxiety and Depression?" *University of Minnesota Center for Spirituality & Healing*. http://www.takingcharge.csh.umn.edu/manage-health-conditions/anxiety-depression/what-lifestyle-changes-are-recommended-anxiety-and-depre.

Leary, Mark R. and June Price Tangney, eds. *Handbook of Self and Identity*. New York: Guilford Press, 2003.

Leifer, John J. and Lori Lindstrom Leifer. *After You Hear It's Cancer*. Lanham, MD: Rowman & Littlefield, 2015.

Lennon, John. *Double Fantasy Stripped Down*. © 2010 by Capitol. Compact disc.

Lennon, John. *Walls and Bridges*. © 2010 by EMI. Compact disc.

Lewis, Nicola L. and John E. Williams. "Acute Pain Management in Patients Receiving Opioids for Chronic and Cancer Pain." *Continuing Education in Anaesthesia, Critical Care & Pain* 5, no. 4 (2005): 127–129. doi: 10.1093/bjaceaccp/mki034.

Lunenburg, Fred C. "Louder than Words: The Hidden Power of Nonverbal Communication in the Workplace." *International Journal of Scholarly Academic Intellectual Diversity* 12, no. 1 (2010): 1–5.

Lutz, Stacey T. and William G. Huitt. "Information Processing and Memory: Theory and Applications." *Educational Psychology Interactive*. Valdosta, GA: Valdosta State University, 2003. http://www.edpsycinteractive.org/papers/infoproc.pdf.

MacLeod, Rod, Jane Vella-Brincat, and Sandy Macleod. *The Palliative Care Handbook: Guidelines for Clinical Management and Symptom Control*. 7th ed. Sydney, Australia: HammondPress, 2014.

Maiorov, Mikhail and Stefan Spinler. "Practical Framework for Intellectual Property Valuation." In *Intellectual Property in Academia: A Practical Guide for Scientists and Engineers* edited by Nadya Reingand, 47. Boca Raton, FL: CRC Press, 2011.

Maltoni, Marco, Emanuela Scarpi, Marta Rosati, Stefania Derni, Laura Fabbri, Francesca Martini, Dino Amadori, and Oriana Nanni. "Palliative Sedation in End-of-Life Care and Survival: A Systematic Review." *Journal of Clinical Oncology* 30, no. 12 (2012): 1378–1383.

Maranhao, Tulio. *The Interpretation of Dialogue*. Chicago: University of Chicago Press, 1990.

Marx, Groucho. *Groucho and Me*. Boston: Da Capo Press, 1959.

Masao, Abe and Steven Heine, eds. *A Study of Dōgen: His Philosophy and Religion*. Albany, NY: SUNY Press, 1992.

McGrath, C. et al. "Toward a Neuroimaging Treatment Selection Biomarker for Major Depressive Disorder." *JAMA Psychiatry* 70, no. 8 (2013): 821–829. doi: 10.1001/jamapsychiatry.2013.143.

McGregor, Graham. "Intonation and Meaning in Conversation." *Language & Communication* 2, no. 2 (1982): 123–131.

Mehler, Jacques, Josiane Bertoncini, and Michele Barriere. "Infant Recognition of Mother's Voice." *Perception*, 7, no. 5 (1978): 491–497.

Merleau-Ponty, M. *Phenomenology of Perception*. Translated by Colin Smith. London: Routledge, 1962.

Meyer, Thomas J. and Melvin M. Mark. "Effects of Psychosocial Interventions with Adult Cancer Patients: A Meta-Analysis of Randomized Experiments." *Health Psychology* 14, no. 2 (1995): 101–108. http://dx.doi.org/10.1037/0278-6133.14.2.101.

Milazzo, S., S. Lejeune, and E. Ernst. "Laetrile for Cancer: A Systematic Review of the Clinical Evidence." *Supportive Care in Cancer* 15, no. 6 (2007): 532–505. doi: 10.1007/s00520-006-0168-9.

Molassiotis, A. et al. "Use of Complementary and Alternative Medicine in Cancer Patients: A European Survey. *Annals of Oncology* 16, no. 4 (2005): 655–663.

Monin, Joan K. and Richard Schulz. "Interpersonal Effects of Suffering in Older Adult Caregiving Relationships." *Psychology and Aging* 24, no. 3 (2009): 681–695. doi: 10.1037/a0016355.

Monk, Thelonious. *Monk's Dream*. Sony Records, 2002.

Montville, Leigh. *Evel: The High-Flying Life of Evel Knievel: American Showman, Daredevil, and Legend*. New York: Anchor, 2012.

Nead, Kevin T., Greg Gaskin, Cariad Chester, Samuel Swisher-McClure, Nicholas J. Leeper, and Nigam H. Shah. "Androgen Deprivation Therapy and Future Alzheimer's Disease Risk." *Journal of Clinical Oncology* 34, no. 6 (2016): 566–571. doi: 10.1200/JCO.2015.63.6266.

Nhat Hanh, Thich. *No Death, No Fear*. New York: Riverhead, 2002.

———. *The Path of Emancipation*. New Delhi: Full Circle Publishing, 2010.

O'Brien, Barbara. "The Wheel of Life: The Realm of Hungry Ghosts." *About.com*. http://buddhism.about.com/od/tibetandeities/ig/Wheel-of-Life-Gallery/Hungry-Ghosts-Realm.htm.

O'Callaghan, Clare C. "Pain, Music Creativity and Music Therapy in Palliative Care." *American Journal of Hospice & Palliative Care* 13, no. 2 (1996): 43–49.

Olsen, Y. and G. Daumit. "Chronic Pain and Narcotics: A Dilemma for Primary Care." *Journal of General Internal Medicine* 17, no. 3 (2002): 238–240. doi: 10.1046/j.1525–1497.2002.20109.x.

Paivio, Allan. *Mental Representations: A Dual Coding Approach*. New York: Oxford University Press, 1990.

Partin, A. W., M. W. Katlan, E. N. Subong, P. C. Walsh, K. J. Wojno, J. E. Oesterling, P. T. Scardino, and J. D. Pearson. "Combination of Prostate-Specific Antigen, Clinical Stage, and Gleason Score to Predict Pathological Stage of Localized Prostate Cancer: A Multi-Institutional Update." *JAMA* 277, no. 18 (1997): 1445–1451.

Peterson, Gail B. "A Day of Great Illumination: B. F. Skinner's Discovery of Shaping." *Journal of the Experimental Analysis of Behavior* 82, no. 3 (2004): 317–328.

Porro, Carlo A., Patrizia Baraldi, Giuseppe Pagnoni, Marco Serafini, Patrizia Facchin, Marta Maieron, and Paolo Nichelli. "Does Anticipation of Pain Affect

Cortical Nociceptive Systems?" *The Journal of Neuroscience* 22, no. 8 (2002): 3206–3214.

"Prostate Cancer." *NIH Research.* http://report.nih.gov/nihfactsheets/ViewFact Sheet.aspx?csid=60.

Punjani, Neelam Saleem. "Truth Telling to Terminally Ill Patients: To Tell or Not to Tell." *Journal of Clinical Research & Bioethics* 4, no. 4 (2013): 159. doi: 10.4172/2155-9627.1000159.

Rashomon. DVD. Directed by Akira Kurosawa. 1950; Tokyo: The Criterion Collection, 2002.

Reeve, Joanne, Mari Lloyd-Williams, and Chris Dowrick. "Depression in Terminal Illness: The Need for Primary Care-Specific Research." *Family Practice* 24, no. 3 (2007): 263–268. doi: 10.1093/fampra/cmm017.

Reynolds, Janice, Debra Drew, and Colleen Dunwoody. "American Society for Pain Management Nursing Position Statement: Pain Management at the End of Life." August 2013. http://www.aspmn.org/documents/PainManagementat theEndofLife_August2013.pdf.

Rinpoche, Sogyal. *Glimpse After Glimpse: Daily Reflections on Living and Dying.* New York: HarperOne, 1995.

———. *Living Well, Dying Well.* Louisville, CO: Sounds True, 1993. Audiobook.

———. *The Tibetan Book of Living and Dying.* San Francisco: HarperCollins, 2012.

———. *Tibetan Wisdom for Living and Dying.* Louisville, CO: Sounds True, 2006. Audiotape.

Rochigneux, P., Michel Resbeut, Frederique Rousseau, Erwan Bories, Jean-Lu Raoul, Flora Poizat, and Laurence Moureu-Zabotto. "Radio(Chemo)Therapy in Elderly Patients with Esophageal Cancer: A Feasible Treatment with an Outcome Consistent with Younger Patients." *Frontiers in Oncology* 4 (2014). http://dx.doi.org/10.3389/fonc.2014.00100.

Rosenblum, Andrew, Lisa A. Marsch, Herman Joseph, and Russell K. Portenoy. "Opioids and the Treatment of Chronic Pain: Controversies, Current Status, and Future Directions." *Experimental and Clinical Psychopharmacology* 16, no. 5 (2008): 404–416. doi: 10.1037/a0013628.

Sagan, Carl, and Ann Druyan. *The Demon-Haunted World: Science as a Candle in the Dark.* New York: Ballantine Books, 1997.

"San Bruno Gas Explosion News." *ABCNews.* http://abcnews.go.com/topics/news/san-bruno-gas-explosion.htm.

Sandler, Howard M., Rodney L. Dunn, P. William McLaughlin, James A. Hayman, Molly A. Sullivan, and Jeremy M. G. Taylor. "Overall Survival After Prostate-Specific-Antigen-Detected Recurrence Following Conformal Radiation Therapy." *International Journal of Radiation Oncology* 48, no. 3 (2000): 629–633.

Sarno, John E. *The Mindbody Prescription: Healing the Body, Healing the Pain.* New York: Warner Books, 1999.

Schachtman, Todd R. and Steve S. Reilly. *Associative Learning and Conditioning Theory: Human and Non-Human Applications.* New York: Oxford University Press, 2011.

Schacter, Daniel L., ed. *How Minds, Brains, and Societies Reconstruct the Past*. Boston: Harvard University Press, 1997.

Schiller, David, ed. *The Little Zen Companion*. New York: Workman Publishing, 1994.

Schneider C., Steven H. Yale, and M. Larson. "Principles of Pain Management." *Clinical Medicine & Research* 1, no. 4 (2003): 337–340.

Seminowicz, D. and Karen D. Davis. "Interactions of Pain Intensity and Cognitive Load: The Brain Stays on Task." *Cerebral Cortex* 17, no. 6 (2007): 1412–1422. doi: 10.1093/cercor/bhl052.

Shah, R. "Current Perspectives on the Gleason Grading of Prostate Cancer." *Archives of Pathology & Laboratory Medicine* 133, no. 11 (2009): 1810–1816.

Shakespeare, William. *History of Richard II*. OpenSource Shakespeare, Act IV, Scene 1. http://www.opensourceshakespeare.org/views/plays/play_view.php?WorkID=richard2&Act=4&Scene=1&Scope=sceneh.

Shakespeare, William. *The Merchant of Venice*. New York: Simon & Schuster, 2009.

Shen, Zhiyuan. "Genomic Instability and Cancer: An Introduction." *Journal of Molecular Cell Biology* 3, no. 1 (2011): 1–3.

"Side Effects of Hormone Therapy." *Prostate Cancer Foundation*. http://www.pcf.org/site/c.leJRIROrEpH/b.5836631/k.3CD9/Side_Effects_of_Hormone_Therapy.htm.

Simons, J. "Prostate Cancer Immunotherapy: Beyond Immunity to Curability." *Cancer Immunology Research* 2, no. 11 (2014): 1034–1043.

Siveke, Ida, Christian Leibold, Evelyn Schiller, and Benedikt Grothe. "Adaptation of Binaural Processing in the Adult Brainstem Induced by Ambient Noise." *The Journal of Neuroscience* 32, no. 2 (2012): 462–473. doi: 10.1523/JNEUROSCI.2094-11.2012.

Skinner, B. F. *Science and Human Behavior*. New York: Free Press, 1965.

Smith, G. Davey and S. Ebrahim, eds. "Hormone Replacement Therapy (HRT): Risks and Benefits." *International Journal of Epidemiology* 30, no. 3 (2001): 423–426.

Snedeker, Jesse and John Trueswell. "Using Prosody to Avoid Ambiguity: Effects of Speaker Awareness and Referential Context." *Journal of Memory and Language* [Internet] 48 (2003): 103–130.

Sprenger, Christian, Falk Eippert, Jürgen Finsterbusch, Ulrike Bingel, Michael Rose, and Christian Büchel. "Attention Modulates Spinal Cord Responses to Pain." *Current Biology* 22, no. 11 (2012): 1019–1022. doi: 10.1016/j.cub.2012.04.006.

Staal, Mark A. "Stress, Cognition, and Human Performance: A Literature Review and Conceptual Framework." Ames Research Center, Moffett Field, California. NASA/TM—2004-212824, 2004. http://human-factors.arc.nasa.gov/flight-cognition/Publications/IH_054_Staal.pdf.

Stark, J. R., S. Perner, M. J. Stamper, J. A. Sinnott, S. Finn, A. S. Eisentein, J. Ma, M. Fiorentino, T. Kurth, M. Loda, E. L. Giovannucci, and L. A. Mucci. "Gleason Score and Lethal Prostate Cancer: Does 3 + 4 = 4 + 3?" *Journal of Clinical Oncology* 27, no. 21 (2009): 3459–3464.

"Statistics and Outlook for Oesophageal Cancer." *Cancer Research UK*. http://www.cancerresearchuk.org/about-cancer/type/oesophageal-cancer/treatment/statistics-and-outlook-for-oesophageal-cancer.

Tang, Siew Tzuh and Shiu-Yu C. Lee. "Cancer Diagnosis and Prognosis in Taiwan: Patient Preferences Versus Experiences." *Psycho-Oncology* 13, no. 1 (2004): 1–13.

The Dalai Lama. *An Open Heart: Practicing Compassion in Everyday Life*. New York: Back Bay Books, 2002.

The Dalai Lama. *The Art of Happiness: A Handbook for Living*. 10th anniversary ed. New York: Riverhead, 2009.

The Wizard of Oz. DVD. Directed by Victor Fleming, George Cukor, Mervyn LeRoy, King Vidor, and Norman Taurog. 1939; Burbank, CA: Warner Home Video, 2000.

Turner, Jane and Brian Kelly, "Emotional Dimensions of Chronic Disease." *Western Journal of Medicine* 172, no. 2 (2000): 124–128.

"Types of Cancer Treatments and Care." *U.S. Food and Drug Administration*. Last updated 6/19/15. http://www.fda.gov/forpatients/illness/cancer/ucm408053.htm.

"Types of Treatment." *National Cancer Institute*. http://www.cancer.gov/about cancer/treatment/types.

Ueda, Makoto. *Basho and His Interpreters*. Stanford, CA: Stanford University Press, 1995.

Uttam, S., H. V. Pham, J. LaFace, B. Leibowitz, J. Yu, R. E. Brand, D. J. Hartman, and Y. Liu. "Early Prediction of Cancer Progression by Depth-Resolved Nanoscale Maps of Nuclear Architecture From Unstained Tissue Specimens." *Cancer Research* 75, no. 22 (2015): 4718–4727.

van Delden, Johannes J. M. "Terminal Sedation: Source of a Restless Ethical Debate." *Journal of Medical Ethics* 33, no. 4 (2007): 187–188.

van der Filler, W. M. and P. Scheltens. "Epidemiology and Risk Factors of Dementia." *Journal of Neurology, Neurosurgery & Psychiatry* 76, no. 5 (2005): 2–7. doi: 10.1136/jnnp.2005.082867.

Varvogli, Liza and Christina Darviri. "Stress Management Techniques: Evidence-Based Procedures That Reduce Stress and Promote Health." *Health Science Journal* 5, no. 2 (2011): 74–89.

Warren, Rick. "The Purpose of Redemptive Suffering." *Daily Hope with Rick Warren*. http://rickwarren.org/devotional/english/the-purpose-of-redemptive-suffering.

"W. C. Fields Biography." *IMDb*. http://www.imdb.com/name/nm0001211/bio.

Weil, Andrew. "Did Steve Jobs Get Good Cancer Treatment?" *DrWeil.com*, http://www.drweil.com/drw/u/QAA401029/Did-Steve-Jobs-Get-Good-Cancer-Treatment.html.

Welz, Stefan, Maximilian Nyazi, Claus Belka, and Ute Ganswindt. "Surgery vs. Radiotherapy in Localized Prostate Cancer: Which Is Best?" *Radiation Oncology* 3, no. 23 (2008): 3–23.

"World Cancer Day 2013—Global Press Release." *worldcancerday.org*. http://www .worldcancerday.org/world-cancer-day-2013-global-press-release.

Zeldan, F., K. T. Martucci, R. A. Kraft, J. G. McHaffie, and R. C. Coghill. "Neural Correlates of Mindfulness Meditation-Related Anxiety Relief." *Social Cognitive and Affective Neuroscience* 9, no. 6 (2013): 751–759. doi: 10.1093/scan/nst041.

Ziemer, Rodger E. and William H. Tranter. *Principles of Communications: Systems Modulation and Noise*. 5th ed. San Francisco: Wiley, 2001.

Zur, Ofer. "Power in Psychotherapy and Counseling: Exploring the 'Inherent Power Differential' and Related Myths About Therapists' Omnipotence and Clients' Vulnerability." *Independent Practitioner* 29, no. 3 (2002): 160–164.

INDEX